ICU Care of Abdominal Organ Transplant Patients

Pittsburgh Critical Care Medicine Series

ICU Care of Abdominal Organ Transplant Patients

Edited by

Ali Al-Khafaji, MD, MPH

Associate Professor of Critical Care Medicine
Department of Critical Care Medicine
University of Pittsburgh School of Medicine
Director, Abdominal Organ Transplant Intensive Care Unit
University of Pittsburgh Medical Center
Pittsburgh, Pennsylvania

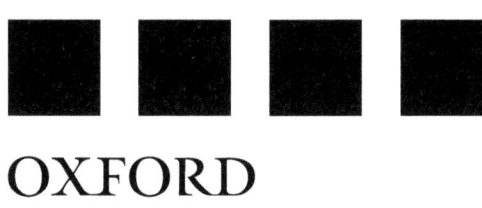

OXFORD
UNIVERSITY PRESS

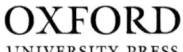

OXFORD

UNIVERSITY PRESS

Oxford University Press is a department of the University of Oxford.
It furthers the University's objective of excellence in research, scholarship,
and education by publishing worldwide.

Oxford   New York
Auckland   Cape Town   Dar es Salaam   Hong Kong   Karachi
Kuala Lumpur   Madrid   Melbourne   Mexico City   Nairobi
New Delhi   Shanghai   Taipei   Toronto

With offices in
Argentina   Austria   Brazil   Chile   Czech Republic   France   Greece
Guatemala   Hungary   Italy   Japan   Poland   Portugal   Singapore
South Korea   Switzerland   Thailand   Turkey   Ukraine   Vietnam

Oxford is a registered trade mark of Oxford University Press in the UK
and certain other countries.

Published in the United States of America by
Oxford University Press
198 Madison Avenue, New York, NY 10016

Library of Congress Cataloging-in-Publication Data
ICU care of abdominal organ transplant patients / editor, Ali Al-Khafaji.
    p. ; cm. — (Pittsburgh critical care medicine series)
Includes bibliographical references and index.
ISBN 978–0–19–976889–9 (alk. paper)
    I. Al-Khafaji, Ali.   II. Series: Pittsburgh critical care medicine.
    [DNLM: 1. Liver Transplantation.   2. End Stage Liver Disease—therapy.   3. Intensive
Care.   4. Kidney Transplantation.   5. Pancreas Transplantation.   6. Perioperative
Care. WI 770]
    617.9′54028—dc23
    2012033697

ISBN 978–0–19–976889–9

9 8 7 6 5 4 3 2 1
Printed in the United States of America
on acid-free paper

I dedicate this book to my late grandmother, Nazhet.
To my parents who instilled the love of medicine in me.
To the love of my life, my wife Dr. Su Min Cho.
Finally to my children, Nazhet and Amir, who keep me going every day.

Series Preface

No place in the world is more closely identified with Critical Care Medicine than Pittsburgh. In the late 1960s, Peter Safar and Ake Grenvik pioneered the science and practice of critical care not just in Pittsburgh but around the world. Their multidisciplinary team approach became the standard for how ICU care is delivered in Pittsburgh to this day. The Pittsburgh Critical Care Medicine series honors this tradition. Edited and largely authored by University of Pittsburgh faculty, the content reflects best practice in critical care medicine. The Pittsburgh model has been adopted by many programs around the world, and local leaders are recognized as world leaders. It is our hope that through this series of concise handbooks, a small part of this tradition can be passed on to the many practitioners of critical care the world over.

John A. Kellum
Series Editor

Preface

When I was approached by Dr. John Kellum to write this book, I was a little hesitant. What could I possibly add to the field by writing this book? There are so many excellent books in critical care, anesthesia, gastroenterology, and transplantation surgery. After initial thought, I concluded that writing a book that takes readers through the long journey of intensive patient care management of multiple medical and surgical problems before and after transplant would be a valuable addition to the critical care literature.

With advances in technology and organization of health-care delivery, many patients with end-stage liver disease that used to die before they could receive a liver transplant now can be supported and managed until they receive the definitive therapy of liver transplantation. Immunosuppressed patients behave differently than other critically ill patients. The delicate balance between over- and underuse of immunosuppressant can lead to significant complications and negative consequences related to rejection, on one extreme, to multiple infections and organ dysfunction on the other end.

The book is divided to two sections. Section 1 (Chapters 1–7) provides a practical and detailed guide on how to manage patients when they present with complications related to end-stage liver disease. Section 2 (Chapters 8–23) addresses the peri-operative management of abdominal organ transplant patients. It provides a very detailed and practical discussion regarding steps taken in addressing the management of every possible complication that can be encountered.

Since Dr Thomas Starzl's arrival at the University of Pittsburgh and the start of the transplant program here, the relationship between the transplant surgeons and the intensivists has continued to flourish so that intensivists have become an integral part of a multidisciplinary team caring for these special patients. Contributors to this book are authorities in their specialties who have put their wealth of knowledge, clinical experience, and practice on paper. Some of the recommendations in this book are not evidence-based for the simple reason that evidence is lacking. I am very grateful to all of them for putting the "Pittsburgh way" in writing to be shared with readers.

I hope this book will be a valuable practical reference for clinicians and students, junior or senior, in the specialties of critical care, gastroenterology, anesthesiology, and transplantation surgery.

Ali Al-Khafaji
2012

Acknowledgments

I am grateful to all my patients who have taught me humility·and an understanding that although our ability as doctors to heal is limited, our capacity for compassion is not. I would like to acknowledge all the nurses and the doctors in the Abdominal Organs Transplant Intensive Care Unit, who are the backbone of our successful transplant critical care program. Special thanks to Dr. David T. Huang for his continued help and input. Finally, I could not have done this without the guidance and constant support from Dr. John Kellum, to whom I will always be grateful.

Contents

Contributors

Ali Abdullah, MD
Department of Anesthesiology
University of Pittsburgh
   Medical
Center Pittsburgh, Pennsylvania

Ali Al-Khafaji, MD, MPH
Associate Professor of Critical Care
   Medicine
Department of Critical Care
   Medicine
University of Pittsburgh School of
   Medicine
Director, Abdominal Organ
   Transplant Intensive Care Unit
University of Pittsburgh Medical
   Center
Pittsburgh, Pennsylvania

Kareem Abu-Elmagd, MD, PhD
Professor of Surgery
Director of the Intestinal
   Rehabilitation and Transplantation
   Center
University of Pittsburgh Medical
   Center
Pittsburgh, Pennsylvania

Christie Bayer, RN, BSN
Abdominal Organ Transplant
   Intensive Care Unit
University of Pittsburgh Medical
   Center
Pittsburgh, Pennsylvania

Deanna Blisard, MD
Department of Critical Care
   Medicine
University of Pittsburgh Medical
   Center
Pittsburgh, Pennsylvania

Charles Boucek, MD
Associate Professor
Department of Anesthesiology
   University of Pittsburgh School of
   Medicine
Pittsburgh, Pennsylvania

Abhideep Chaudhary, MD
University of Pittsburgh Medical
   Center
Pittsburgh, Pennsylvania

Su Min Cho, MD, MRCP
Division of Gastroenterology,
   Hepatology, and Nutrition
University of Pittsburgh School of
   Medicine
Pittsburgh, Pennsylvania

Kapil B. Chopra, MD
Associate Professor of Medicine
Director of Hepatology
Medical Director, Liver
   Transplantation
Medical Director, Comprehensive
   Liver Program, UPMC Liver
   Pancreas Ins
Director, Transplant Hepatology
   Fellowship Program
Division of Gastroenterology,
   Hepatology, and Nutrition
University of Pittsburgh School of
   Medicine
Pittsburgh, Pennsylvania

Guilherme Costa, MD, FACS
Assistant Professor
General Surgery Residency Program
University of Pittsburgh Medical
   Center
Pittsburgh, Pennsylvania

Matthew Cove, MD

Department of Critical Care Medicine
University of Pittsburgh Medical
    Center
Pittsburgh, Pennsylvania

Susan DeRubis

MS, RN, CCRN
Transplant Intensive Care Unit
University of Pittsburgh Medical
    Center
Pittsburgh, Pennsylvania

Rebecca Gooch, MD

Department of Critical Care
    Medicine
University of Pittsburgh Medical
    Center
Pittsburgh, Pennsylvania

Tracy Grogan, RN, BSN, CCRN

Director, Abdominal Organ
    Transplant Intensive Care Unit
University of Pittsburgh Medical
    Center
Pittsburgh, Pennsylvania

Jana G. Hashash, MD

Division of Gastroenterology,
    Hepatology, and Nutrition
University of Pittsburgh School of
    Medicine
Pittsburgh, Pennsylvania

**Richard J. Hendrickson, MD,
FACS, FAAP**

Associate Professor of Pediatrics
University of Missouri-Kansas City
    School of Medicine
Kansas City, Missouri

Ibtesam Hilmi, MD, FRCA

Associate Professor
Department of Anesthesiology
University of Pittsburgh Medical
    Center
Pittsburgh, Pennsylvania

Abhinav Humar MD

Professor
Department of Surgery
University of Pittsburgh School of
    Medicine and
Chief of Transplantation
University of Pittsburgh Medical
    Center
Pittsburgh, Pennsylvania

Prem A. Kandiah, MD

Department of Critical Care
    Medicine
University of Pittsburgh Medical
    Center
Pittsburgh, Pennsylvania

Michael C Koprucki, MD

Division of General Internal Medicine
University of Pittsburgh Medical
    Center
Pittsburgh, Pennsylvania

Ahmad Maarouf, MD

Department of Critical Care Medicine
University of Pittsburgh Medical
    Center
Pittsburgh, Pennsylvania

Jerry McAuley, MD

Professor of Medicine, Department
    of Medicine
Professor of Surgery, Department of
    Surgery
Director, Transplant Nephrology,
    UPMC Transplantation Institute
Medical Director, Kidney/Pancreas
    Transplantation
University of Pittsburgh Medical
    Center
Pittsburgh, Pennsylvania

Juan Mejia, MD

Fellow, Transplantation Surgery
University of Pittsburgh Medical
    Center
Pittsburgh, Pennsylvania

Thiruvengadam Muniraj, MD
Department of Internal Medicine
Mercy Hospital of Pittsburgh
Pittsburgh, Pennsylvania

M. Hong Nguyen, MD
Professor of Medicine
Director, Transplant Infectious
    Diseases
Director, Antimicrobial Management
    Program
University of Pittsburgh Medical
    Center
Pittsburgh, Pennsylvania

Stephen O'Keefe, MD
Professor of Medicine
Medical Director, Small Intestinal
    Rehabilitation & Transplant
    Center
Division of Gastroenterology,
    Hepatology, and Nutrition
University of Pittsburgh School of
    Medicine
Pittsburgh, Pennsylvania

Federico Palacio, MD
University of Texas Health Sciences
San Antonio, Texas
and
The University of Pittsburgh
Pittsburgh, Pennsylvania

Raymond Planinsic, MD
Professor of Anesthesiology
Director of Transplantation
    Anesthesiology
University of Pittsburgh School of
    Medicine
Pittsburgh, Pennsylvania

**Jose Renan da Cunha-Melo,
MD, PhD**
General Surgery & Digestive Tract
    Surgery
Hospital das Clinicas UFMG

Ely M. Sebastian, MD
Center for Organ Transplantation
Our Lady of Lourdes Medical Center
Camden, New Jersey

Faraaz Shah, MD
Assistant Professor of Medicine
Renal-Electrolyte Division
University of Pittsburgh School of
    Medicine
Pittsburgh, Pennsylvania

Ron Shapiro, MD
Professor of Surgery
University of Pittsburgh School of
    Medicine
Pittsburgh, Pennsylvania

Kate Foryt, RN, CCRN
Abdominal Organ Transplant
    Intensive Care Unit
University of Pittsburgh Medical Center
Pittsburgh, Pennsylvania

Martin Wijkstrom, MD
Assistant professor of surgery
division of transplantation surgery
University of Pittsburgh Medical
    center
Pittsburgh, Pennsylvania

Sachin Yende, MD MS
Associate Professor
Director of CRISMA Research
    Fellowship
Department of Critical Care Medicine
University of Pittsburgh Medical
    Center
Pittsburgh, Pennsylvania

Section 1

Intensive Care Unit Management of Patients With Decompensated Liver Disease

The onset of complications related to end-stage liver disease (ESLD) defines the transition from a compensated to decompensated state, which carries worse morbidity and mortality. Critically ill patients with ESLD admitted to the intensive care unit (ICU) have an overall mortality rate ranging from 50% to 100%. Patients with ESLD usually are referred for transplantation evaluation when their model for ESLD scores are 10 or they have a major complication develop that is related to liver disease, such as hepatic encephalopathy or variceal bleeding. Patients with ESLD admitted to the ICU who are not candidates for liver transplantation have a particularly poor long-term prognosis, even if they survive the ICU admission. In this section, there will be a discussion of the specific ESLD complications and its management.

Selected reference

Al-Khafaji A & Huang DT. Critical care management of patients with end-stage liver disease. *Crit Care Med.* 2011;39(5):1157–1166.

Chapter 1

Spontaneous Bacterial Peritonitis

Su Min Cho and Ali Al-Khafaji

Patients with end-stage liver disease (ESLD) have significant immune dysfunction, higher rates of infection, and sepsis. Any infection likely worsens liver function *per se*, including contributing to risk of variceal bleeding. Spontaneous bacterial peritonitis (SBP) is the most common infection in patients with ESLD and can precipitate decompensation. Spontaneous bacterial peritonitis can present with no or vague symptoms, and clinical examination alone cannot exclude SBP.

Paracentesis should be routinely performed in critically ill patients suffering from ESLD with ascites. Most clinicians use an ascitic fluid polymorphonuclear (PMN) count of > 250 cells/uL as the standard diagnostic cut-off for SBP.

White blood cell count > 1000 cells/uL, pH < 7.35, or blood-ascitic fluid pH gradient > 0.1 can be used as an alternative cut-offs.

Concomitant blood cultures should also be drawn because bacteremia is present in approximately half of SBP cases and can help identify the organism.

Culture-negative neutrocytic ascites (polymorphonuclear ≥ 250 cells/uL but culture negative) and bacterascites (polymorphonuclear < 250 cells/uL but culture-positive) should be treated the same as SBP.

Antibiotic coverage should be directed at Gram–negative aerobic bacteria (*Escherichia coli, Klebsiella pneumoniae*) and Gram–positive cocci (*Streptococcus, Enterococci*).

Third-generation cephalosporins are most commonly recommended, but unit antibiograms and individual patient antibiotic exposure history also should be considered. Although controversial, albumin reduced mortality in one trial, whereas a recent observational study suggested albumin may only benefit patients with SBP with elevated creatinine, blood urea nitrogen, or total bilirubin.

It is well accepted that patients presenting with acute gastrointestinal bleeding should receive empirical antibiotics because such patients are at high risk for SBP, and occult SBP can precipitate gastrointestinal bleeding. Secondary bacterial peritonitis should be considered if ascitic fluid shows a polymorphonuclear count in the thousands, multiple organisms, or elevated protein levels. Lack of clinical improvement despite empirical antibiotics should prompt consideration of abdominal imaging and a repeat paracentesis to look for resistant organisms, secondary bacterial peritonitis, or both.

In one study, patients with SBP had higher Child-Pugh and model for ESLD scores at the time of transplantation compared with controls, but there was no difference in long-term mortality between the two groups. Patients with SBP, however, were more likely to require surgery for complications related to LT within 1 year and were more likely to die of sepsis.

Selected references

Rimola A, Garcia-Tsao G, Navasa M, et al. Diagnosis, treatment and prophylaxis of spontaneous bacterial peritonitis: A consensus document. *International Ascites Club. J Hepatol* 2000;32:142–153.

Chapter 2

Hepatic Encephalopathy

Prem A. Kandiah, Thiruvengadam Muniraj, and Ali Al-Khafaji

Introduction

Hepatic encephalopathy (HE) is a term used in the clinical setting to describe a wide spectrum of neuropsychiatric deficits associated with acute liver failure, chronic liver failure, or the presence of a portosystemic shunt. In acute liver failure, HE charts a more lethal course characterized by progression into coma, intracranial hypertension, and cerebral herniation. In patients with end-stage liver disease (ESLD) or cirrhosis, the onset is more insidious, with an expansive repertoire of cognitive and motor deficits. Early symptoms of this syndrome include reversal of sleep patterns, apathy, hypersomnia, irritability, and personal neglect. In later stages, delirium and coma can arise with neurological signs, including asterixis, hyperreflexia, rigidity, and myoclonus.

The two major classifications systems for HE include the consensus terminology by the World congress of Gastroenterology and the West Haven Criteria (Tables 2.1 and 2.2). Although these findings in ESLD are generally thought to be reversible, there is growing body of evidence suggesting an element of persistent cognitive and motor deficits implicating a degenerative process in patients with severe HE. Pre-transplant HE was associated with post-liver transplant neurocognitive deficits, suggesting that some level of irreversible injury is attributable to HE. A fraction of patients with chronic liver disease with rapidly deteriorating liver function (acute-on-chronic liver failure) have been reported to develop intracranial hypertension, which is more characteristic for acute liver failure. This suggests that the pathogenesis of HE-associated cerebral edema for any acute liver injury is independent of chronicity. Hepatic encephalopathy in patients with cirrhosis is considered a poor prognostic sign; without liver transplantation, the 1-year survival rate is 42% after the first episode of overt HE, and the 3-year survival rate is 23%.

Pathophysiology

There is no single clear etiology accounting for the occurrence of HE. There is, however, some evidence to suggest that HE is a result of a complex interplay

Table 2.1 Classification of Hepatic Encephalopathy by the World Congress of Gastroenterology

Classification	Underlying hepatic or extra-hepatic etiology
Type A	Acute liver failure
Type B	Portosystemic bypass without intrinsic hepato-cellular damage
Type C	Cirrhosis and portal hypertension with portal-systemic shunts

Table 2.2 West Haven Criteria for Grading Severity Hepatic Encephalopathy

Classification	Symptom characteristics and physical findings
Minimal encephalopathy	Minimal changes in memory evident of psychometric testing. Absence of detectable changes in personality and behavior.
Grade 1	Trivial lack of awareness; euphoria or anxiety; shortened attention span; impaired performance of addition or subtraction
Grade 2	Lethargy or apathy; minimal disorientation for time or place; subtle personality change; inappropriate behavior; asterixsis usually present.
Grade 3	Somnolence to semi-stupor but responsive to verbal stimuli; confusion; gross disorientation; clonus; nystagmus; positive Babinski sign
Grade 4	Grade 4–Coma (unresponsive to verbal or noxious stimuli); dysconjugate eye movements, ocular bobbing, decorticate and decerebrate posturing may be present.

among brain ammonia, inflammation, altered neurotransmission pathways, and cerebral hemodynamic dysautoregulation. Hyperammonemia continues to play a central role in the development of HE.

Ammonia is thought to result in both cytotoxic and vasogenic brain edema caused by the cerebral energy failure, excessive intracellular accumulation of the osmolyte glutamine, and alterations in aquaporin-4 integral membrane proteins. A plasma ammonia level of more than 150 µmol/L is associated with an increased risk of cerebral edema and brain herniation in acute liver failure (ALF). Cerebral edema in HE is thought to be a combination of both a vasogenic and cytotoxic process. The contributive role of inflammation, altered neurotransmission pathways, and cerebral hemodynamic dysautoregulation may, in part, explain the presence of HE in some patients with a relatively low serum ammonia level.

Ammonia Homeostasis

The bowel governs the production of ammonia, and the liver facilitates clearance of excess glutamine and ammonia via the urea cycle. The kidney, in turn, produces or clears ammonia depending on multiple circumstances and has recently been shown to play a more significant role in the production of ammonia in diseased state. Although muscle and brain have the capacity to detoxify large amounts of ammonia to glutamine, they remain dependent on the liver and kidney to clear excess glutamine. Anabolic homeostasis incorporates excess circulating glutamine into protein building; however, this is seldom the case in the acutely ill intensive care unit (ICU) patient, whereby catabolism further contributes to the glutamine load, which is a precursor to ammonia. Current ammonia-lowering therapeutic strategies in HE are targeted at various points along this pathway to augment clearance or to decrease production of ammonia.

Diagnosis

Hepatic encephalopathy is a diagnosis of exclusion requiring a detailed history, physical exam, and laboratory investigation. Similar neuropsychiatric symptoms may be seen in various other metabolic processes, toxic ingestion or drug overdoses, infectious processes, or intracranial processes. In patients with cirrhosis and portosystemic shunting, a known precipitating factor and a typical clinical presentation is usually sufficient to make a clinical diagnosis. The presence of elevated serum ammonia is helpful, as it does correlate with severity of HE; however, absence of a significant elevation in serum ammonia does not rule out HE.

Prompt recognition of the precipitating factors also helps delineate the approach to treatment. Eighty percent of patients with HE have precipitating factors, which are reversible. Table 2.3 lists the common precipitating factors and underlying mechanism in HE. Laboratory testing is necessary to exclude treatable causes such as hypoxia, azotemia, hyponatremia, hypoglycemia, and psychoactive drugs or toxins. Further work-up including EEG, brain imaging, and lumbar puncture may be necessary, especially in the presence of less typical features such as seizures or focal or lateralizing neurological deficits on exam. The physical exam can be challenging in grade 4 encephalopathy, where dysconjugate eye movements, ocular bobbing, and decorticate and decerebrate posturing may be present, making it difficult to differentiate from an intracranial process. There have been reported cases of reversible focal deficits coinciding with severe HE. The possibility of a subdural hemorrhage needs to be considered, especially in patients with alcoholic cirrhosis who may sustain falls. Finally, the diagnosis of minimal HE can only be made by psychometric tests and is not reviewed here, as it has less of a role in the ICU setting.

Treatment

To date, there remains no robust clinical evidence to effectively guide clinicians in the management of HE using the existing armamentarium. In the ICU setting, the approach to management HE is aimed at:

1. Treatment of precipitating factors in parallel with intensive care supportive strategies

Table 2.3 Precipitating Factors and Underlying Mechanisms in Hepatic Encephalopathy

Mechanism	Precipitating factor
Excess Extra-portal Nitrogen Burden	• Gastrointestinal bleed • Blood transfusions • Infection • Constipation • Azotemia • Starvation • Excess dietary protein • Portosystemic shunt (iatrogenic and spontaneous)
Impaired toxin Clearance	• Dehydration caused by excessive fluid restriction, excessive diuresis or paracentesis, diarrhea • Hypotension resulting from bleeding or systemic vasodilatation • Abdominal Compartment syndrome caused by severe ascites
Altered neurotransmission	• Benzodiazepine use • Coinciding alcohol withdrawal • Psychoactive drugs
Acute hepatocellular damage	• Alcoholic hepatitis • Drugs • Acute viral hepatitis • Development of hepatocellular carcinoma

II. Initiation of HE specific therapeutic strategies
1. Reduction of intestinal ammonia production and absorption
2. Plasma ammonia-lowering devices and nonpharmacological interventions
3. Alternative pathway therapies
4. Neurotransmitter blockade
5. Nutritional and micronutrient supplementation

Neurological System

- Although the West Haven Criteria is a well-accepted method to broadly categorize severity of encephalopathy, the severity of encephalopathy quickly escalates to grade 3 and grade 4 in the ICU setting. The Glasgow coma scale is a useful grading system to monitor the level of consciousness in patients with grade 3 and grade 4 encephalopathy, especially because it is a commonly used tool by nurses in ICUs.
- Avoid sedatives when possible. Avoid intermediate and long-acting benzodiazepines at all times because of decreased clearance by the liver. For intubated patients, Propofol would be the sedative of choice.

- Occasionally, alcohol withdrawal and HE can coexist. Symptom-triggered therapy with lorazepam may be tried with caution. Intubation for airway protection, use of propofol for sedation, and management of alcohol withdrawal would be the next option.
- Intracranial hypertension is uncommon in ESLD; however, a small subset of patients with acute-on-chronic liver failure will develop intracranial hypertension and brain herniation. There is no clear predictive evidence to determine who will develop intracranial hypertension. However, patients with no significant baseline cortical atrophy are thought to be most at risk. These typically include younger patients with non-alcoholic cirrhosis in persistent grade 4 encephalopathy with evidence of acutely deteriorating liver function.

Respiratory System

- Anticipate deterioration in mental status if a HE precipitating factor is not resolved (e.g., variceal bleed). Early elective intubation in this scenario would avoid a more complicated emergent intubation and possibly reduce the occurrence of aspiration.

Cardiovascular System

- Sepsis is frequently the underlying precipitating factor in HE, and it is often difficult to differentiate hypotension because of sepsis or a vasodilatory state resulting from early liver failure. Using the early goal-directed therapy for sepsis algorithm is an appropriate way to begin managing the hemodynamic status.

Renal System and Electrolytes

- Optimal renal function is crucial to the management of hyperammonemia. In transplant candidates, consider early use of continuous renal replacement therapy (CRRT) if the patient has refractory hyperammonemia in the presence of significant acute kidney injury or hepatorenal syndrome.
- Hypokalemia and metabolic acidosis increases renal ammonia production. Anecdotal evidence links hyponatremia to progression of cerebral edema in chronic liver failure. Metabolic alkalosis promotes formation of (NH_3^+) that crosses the blood–brain barrier from (NH_4^+).

Gastrointestinal System and Nutrition

- Control bleeding early. Anticipate worsening encephalopathy during and after active gastrointestinal bleeding (GIB).

- The use of antibiotics in GIB reduces infections and improves short-term survival.
- Consider early transjugular intrahepatic portosystemic shunt (TIPS) placement in patients in addition to endoscopic band ligation.
- In the event TIPS is performed, anticipate possible deterioration in grade of HE. This is usually transient and self-limiting. Monitoring serum ammonia levels pre- and post-TIPS with the timely use of ammonia-lowering agents may help reduce the severity of encephalopathy.
- Constipation should be managed with lactulose (oral or enema), which remains the mainstay of therapy in patients with HE. The goal is to achieve at least two bowel movements per day. If the goal is not achieved, then consider polyethylene glycol electrolyte solution (Golytely®) via nasogastric tube and enema.
- Protein restriction promotes catabolism, which fuels ammoniagenesis and therefore should be avoided. An enteric formula approximating 30 kcal/kg/day containing a 3:1 ratio of carbohydrate to fat with addition of 1.2 g/kg/day of protein is appropriate with HE. Actual body weight is difficult to determine in late stages of cirrhosis because of coexisting edema and ascites; therefore, ideal body weight should be used to calculate enteric formula.

Endocrine System

- Hypoglycemia is common in a failing liver and cannot be clinically detected in grade 4 encephalopathy. Hypoglycemia potentially worsens liver failure and brain edema. Serial blood glucose monitoring is important in later stages of HE.

Infection, Hematologic, and Immune System

- Obtain appropriate cultures and initiate broad spectrum antibiotics early. Spontaneous bacterial peritonitis occurs in 8% to 30% of hospitalized cirrhotic patients with ascites and needs to be excluded. Early use of antibiotics improves outcome. De-escalation of antibiotics is appropriate based on the clinical picture and culture results.

Initiation of Hepatic Encephalopathy-Specific Therapeutic Strategies

1. Reduction of intestinal ammonia production and absorption
   i. Lactulose (β-galactosidofructose) and Lactitol (β-galactosidosorbitol)
      Both these nonabsorbable disaccharides are currently first-line agents for the treatment of HE. However, neither drug has been shown thus far to improve mortality.

Mechanism of Action:

i. Lactulose is converted to Lactid acid and Acetic acid, resulting in acidification of gut lumen. This favors conversion of NH_3^+ to NH_4^+, which is relatively membrane-impermeable and less absorbed.

ii. Gut acidification inhibits ammoniagenic coliform bacteria, leading to increased levels of nonammoniagenic lactobacilli.

iii. As a cathartic agent that decreases transit time, lactulose may clear gut ammonia before it can be absorbed.

Dosage:

Oral or via nasogastric tube: 45 mL initially followed by repeated dose every hour until patient has a bowel movement. More appropriate in patients who are alert or intubated with low aspiration risk. Once bowel movement achieved, titrate lactulose (15–45 mL every 8–12 hours) to achieve three soft bowel movements per day. Production of liquid stool should be avoided, as it will worsen the patients' nutritional status and promote further catabolism.

Enema: 300 mL in 700 mL water retained for 1 hour in Trendenlenberg position. More appropriate in patients with grade 3 to 4 encephalopathy where risk of aspiration is high.

ii) AST-120

AST -120 is not FDA approved and is unavailable in the United States. It is a spherical carbon absorbent originally used in Japan to treat uremic pruritis. It is nontoxic with the capability of binding ammonia in the gut. Preliminary human studies have demonstrated it to be as effective as lactulose.

2. Ammonia-lowering antibiotics

i. Rifaximin: Recently approved by the FDA for chronic HE, rifaximin is an oral nonsystemic antibiotic with less than 0.4% absorption. A recent multicenter clinical trial in the outpatient setting using Rifaximin at the dose of 550 mg orally twice daily for 6 months in patients with chronic HE offered significant protection against recurrent HE episodes and hospital admissions compared to placebo. For Acute HE grade 1 to 3 rifaximin was shown to be as effective as lactitol in the treatment of grades 1 to 3 HE. Both treatments achieved an efficacy of greater than 80%. In addition, rifaximin showed significantly greater efficacy in the reduction of plasma ammonia levels and improvement in EEG than those observed with lactitol.

ii. Neomycin: FDA approved for the management of Acute HE despite very small and conflicting studies supporting its use. Dosage: 1000 mg every 6 hours for up to 6 days in acute HE. For chronic HE, 1 to 2 grams daily may be used. Despite its poor absorption, chronic administration can result in nephrotoxicity and ototoxicity.

iii. Metronidazole: Not FDA approved for management of HE. One small study revealed it is as effective as Neomycin at a dose of 250 mg twice daily. The concern for resistant Clostridium Difficile colitis and neuro-toxic effects of metronidazole caused by systemic absorption has limited routine use in patients with HE.

3. Plasma ammonia-lowering devices and nonpharmacological interventions
   i. Hemodialysis and continuous renal replacement therapy
      Continuous renal replacement therapy, specifically ultrafiltation, with the use of high dialysate flow rate, is an effective method of rapidly lowering serum plasma ammonia levels. A higher flow rate is achievable with conventional hemodialysis but is less tolerated because of the frequency hemodynamic instability in these patients. In a select few patients, a combination of both could be used. Avoid hemodialysis in patients with suspected intracranial hypertension, as fluid shifts may worsen the cerebral edema.
   ii. Molecular Adsorbent Recirculating System
      Molecular Adsorbent Recirculating System (MARS) is a blood detoxification system based on albumin dialysis that removes protein-bound and water-soluble toxins. The FDA has approved MARS as a toxin removal device in cases of poisoning and overdose but not for HE. In the United States, MARS is used in some centers in the management of acute liver failure caused by drug overdose or toxic exposures. In a randomized, double-blind, multicenter study of patients with cirrhosis with grade 3 and grade 4 HE, the MARS dialysis-treated group had more significant and rapid improvement in their mental status compared to standard medical therapy.

4. Alternative pathway therapy
   i. Sodium benzoate and sodium phenylacetate
      Using an alternative pathway for the metabolism of ammonia, sodium benzoate and sodium phenyl acetate have been shown to enhance the metabolism of ammonia. Both the amino acids glycine and glutamine are nitrogen intermediaries of ammonia. Benzoate conjugates with glycine while phenylacetate conjugates glutamine to form hippuric acid and phenylacetylglutamine, respectively, which can be excreted by the kidneys. At present, Ammonul® (10% sodium benzoate and 10% sodium phenylacetate) is FDA approved and routinely used for the treatment of hyperammonemia in urea cycle disorders. One small study has shown benefit in the treatment of HE. Oral doses of sodium benzoate alone at a dose of 5 g bid was as effective as lactulose in reducing serum ammonia levels in another small study. A significant limitation of both these drugs is its reliance on the good renal function, which is often impaired in cirrhotic patients with multisystem organ failure in the ICU. The only preparation available in the United States, Ammonul®, is very costly compared to the extremely inexpensive preparations of sodium benzoate available in Europe.

ii. L-ornithine L-aspartate (LOLA)
Although intravenous doses of L-ornithine L-aspartate (LOLA) showed promise in multiple small studies at reducing serum ammonia levels and improving encephalopathy, a recent randomized double-blind, placebo-controlled study failed to show an effective ammonia lowering effect or decreased mortality.

iii. Ornithinephenylacetate—Animal studies have demonstrated enhanced conversion of ammonia to glutamine and subsequently trapping it as phenylacetylglutamine, which is excreted by the kidneys. Additional ammonia-lowering effects are thought to come from enhanced muscle glutamine synthetase and normalization of intestinal glutaminase activity.

5. Neurotransmitter blockade
Flumazenil—In a systematic review involving 13 controlled trials with a total of 805 patients, the use of flumazenil was associated with significant improvement in HE but failed to show long-term benefits or improvement in outcome. As a short-acting benzodiazepine antagonist, Flumazenil is postulated to inhibit endogenous GABAergic substances and previous residual effects of long-acting benzodiazepine. Cirrhotics have also been shown to have increased benzodiazepine receptor activation, but only a subset of patients will demonstrate response to Flumazenil. Flumazenil should be used in a closely monitored environment, as it has a potential of provoking seizures.

Dosage: A trial of 1 to 2 mg of Flumazenil in 20 mL saline solution by intravenous infusion for 3 to 5 minutes may be considered in patients with stage 3 to 4 encephalopathy who have low serum ammonia level and have not responded to Lactulose.

6. Nutritional and micronutrient supplementation
Zinc and Carnitine supplementation—There are numerous anecdotal reports and small studies about the ammonia-lowering effects of oral supplementation with Zinc and Carnitine, which requires further study.

Branched-chain amino acid supplementation—Improvement in HE has been noted in patients predominantly treated in the outpatient setting, without improvement in mortality. Its role in the ICU remains unproven.

Selected References

Als-Nielsen B, Gluud LL, Gluud C. Nonabsorbable disaccharides for hepatic encephalopathy: Systematic review of randomized trials. *BMJ* 2004;328:1046

Bass NM, Mullen KD, Sanyal A, et al. Rifaximin treatment in hepatic encephalopathy. *N Engl J Med* 2010;362:1071–1081

Sharma BC, Sharma P, Agrawal A, et al. Secondary prophylaxis of hepatic encephalopathy: An open-label randomized controlled trial of lactulose versus placebo. *Gastroenterology* 2009;137:885–891, e881

Chapter 3

Upper Gastrointestinal Bleeding

S Chandra, Su Min Cho, and Ali Al-Khafaji

Upper gastrointestinal bleeding (UGIB) is a major cause of morbidity and mortality in patients with end-stage liver disease (ESLD) and in majority of the cases is a direct consequence of portal hypertension (PH). Despite improvements in therapeutic options and supportive therapy, the 6-week mortality rate remains high: from 15% to 30% in patients with Child class C. The annual incidence of UGIB in patients with cirrhosis and PH is approximately 25% to 35% per year.

Esophageal and gastric variceal bleeding accounts for the majority of episodes of UGIB in patients with cirrhosis. In a study of 465 patients with cirrhosis, the etiology for UGIB was esophageal varices (64%), gastric varices (8.4%), portal hypertensive gastropathy (9.5%), and peptic ulcer disease (7.5%), with esophagitis, erosions, and esophageal ulcers accounting for the rest.

The management of variceal bleeding is focused on achieving three major goals: prevention of first bleeding episode, management of active bleeding, and prophylaxis of recurrent bleeding.

In our intensive care unit (ICU), all patients with ESLD who present with UGIB will have their airway secured prior to endoscopy to prevent aspiration. This will also give the endoscopist a controlled environment to perform their endoscopic therapy.

Prevention of First Bleeding Episode

The formation of esophageal varices in cirrhotic patients is approximately 7% per year, with the rate being higher for patients with decompensated liver disease. Varices are present in 30% to 40% of patients with compensated liver disease and in 60% of patients with decompensated liver disease at the time of diagnosis. Portal pressure plays a critical role in the formation of varices and hepatic venous pressure gradient (HVPG) of 10 mmHg is considered as threshold for the development of varices.

Variceal hemorrhage occurs at a yearly rate of 5% to 15%, and the predictors for high risk of bleeding include the size of varices, advanced liver disease (Child class B or C), and presence of red wale marks on varices.

- In patients without varices, no prophylactic treatment is recommended.
- In patients with small varices who are at low risk for bleeding (absence of red wale marks and without advanced liver disease), prophylaxis with non-selective beta-blockers may be considered as an option, although there are limited data to support this therapy.
- In patients with small varices who are at high risk for bleeding (presence of red wale marks and advanced liver disease), nonselective beta-blockers are recommended.
- In patients with medium/large varices, nonselective beta-blockers should be considered as the first-choice treatment to prevent first bleeding, whereas esophageal variceal band ligation should be used for patients with contrain-dication or intolerance to beta-blockers.

Management of Active Bleeding

Active UGIB from esophageal varices is a medical emergency with a mortality rate approaching 20% to 30%. The goals for initial management include securing and protecting the airway, hemodynamic stabilization with fluid resuscitation, and blood transfusions followed by directed therapy to control the source of bleeding. Because successful management requires a multidisciplinary team approach, all patients should be managed in the ICU. Patients should be fre-quently assessed for their ability to maintain a patent airway, and patients with encephalopathy and UGIB should have their airway secured. Fluid resuscita-tion and blood transfusion should be aimed at maintaining a systolic pressure of about 100 mmHg and Hgb of around 8 gm/dL. Overzealous volume expansion can potentially cause rebound increase in portal pressure and increased bleed-ing. Although not supported by the literature, correction of coagulopathy is usually done in most institutions, including ours, prior to endoscopy. The use of recombinant factor VII in patients with variceal bleed is not recommended.

Combination of pharmacological therapy with endoscopic band ligation (EBL) therapy remains the most rational approach in the management of acute variceal bleeding.

Vasoactive Drug Therapy

Pharmacological therapy with vasoactive agents is the first line of therapy for the management of an acute variceal bleed, and it should be instituted as soon as the diagnosis of variceal bleeding is suspected and before confirmation with esophagogastroduodenoscopy (EGD). Vasoactive drugs decrease the variceal blood flow by decreasing portal pressure and potentially limit the amount of bleeding. Two classes of drugs are used: vasopressin and its analogs (terlipres-sin) and somatostatin and its analogs (octreotide/vapreotide).

Vasopressin causes reduction in splanchnic blood flow and thus significant decrease in portal pressure. However, its clinical use is limited because of serious side effects caused by cardiac and peripheral vascular ischemia. It should only be used when other drugs are not available and in conjunction with nitroglycerine. Terlipressin is a synthetic analog of vasopressin with longer duration of action and with fewer side effects. It is the only drug that has shown to improve survival, with overall efficacy of controlling variceal bleeding around 67% at 5 days. However, terlipressin can cause ischemic complications and should be avoided in patients with a history of ischemic heart disease, vascular disorders, and rhythm disorders.

Octreotide is a synthetic analog of natural somatostatin with similar mechanism of action and is the only drug approved for the treatment of acute variceal bleed in the United States. Randomized control trials have shown that octreotide may have added benefit if used together with endoscopic therapy but its benefit if used alone is not clear. The duration of pharmacological therapy with vasoactive drugs is generally 5 days, as the risk of rebleeding is highest during this period.

Endoscopic Therapy

Endoscopy is the gold standard of management of active UGI bleeding because it is diagnostic as well as therapeutic and thus should be considered early as soon as initial hemodynamic and airway stabilization is achieved.

The two endoscopic methods available are EBL and endoscopic sclerotherapy (EST).

Endoscopic Band Ligation

The procedure involves placement of elastic bands on the varices which results in its occlusion and thrombosis. The tissue then necroses and sloughs off in a few days to weeks, leaving a superficial mucosal ulceration, which rapidly heals. The complications are rare and include dysphagia, chest pain, bleeding, and infection. More serious complications involve massive bleeding from variceal rupture, bleeding from ulcer, and esophageal strictures.

Sclerotherapy

Endoscopic sclerotherapy was the first endoscopic technique developed for the management of bleeding varices. Sclerotherapy for esophageal varices involves injecting a strong and irritating solution (a sclerosant) into the veins and/or the area beside the distended vein. Ethanolamine or sodium tetradecyl sulphate are used most commonly. The sclerosant causes necrosis, fibrosis, and ultimately obliteration of the varices. Complications with sclerotherapy include esophagitis, stricture formation, and, rarely, perforation.

Although both EBL and EST are proven strategies for control of acute variceal bleeding, EBL is considered by most specialists as the preferred choice for endoscopic management and EST should be considered if EBL is not available.

Rescue Therapies

In 10% to 20% of episodes of acute variceal bleeding, conventional combination therapy of vasoactive drugs and endoscopy fails to control the bleeding. In such cases of refractory bleeding, rescue therapies are employed.

Transjugular Intrahepatic Portosystemic Shunt. Transjugular intrahepatic portosystemic shunt (TIPS) is the formation of a low-resistance conduit between a portal vein and a hepatic vein by deployment of an intrahepatic expandable stent that results in reduction of portal vein pressure. The procedure results in achievement of hemostasis in more than 90% of cases; however, the 6-week mortality remains very high when used as rescue therapy (35%). A recent study has shown the benefits of early TIPS in patients with high risk of bleeding (Child–Pugh Class B with active bleeding at endoscopy or in Child–Pugh Class C). In this study, patients who underwent TIPS within 96 hours of admission after combination therapy (vasoactive drugs + endoscopic therapy) had significant reduction in treatment failure and mortality. This study has exciting implications for the use of TIPS as a first-line therapy for acute variceal bleeding in patients who are at high risk of rebleeding.

Balloon Tamponade. In cases of massive bleeding or failed combination therapy with vasoactive drugs and endoscopy, balloon tamponade offers a temporary attempt at controlling the bleeding and a bridge to either another attempt with endoscopy or TIPS. A double-balloon tamponade tube originally developed by Sengstaken and Blakemore in 1950 consists of a gastric balloon, an esophageal balloon, and a gastric suction port. The addition of an esophageal suction port to help prevent aspiration of esophageal contents resulted in what is called the Minnesota tube. Balloon tamponade initially controls the hemorrhage in 60% to 90% of cases. Balloon tamponade should be only a temporizing measure, before more definitive therapy is instituted. Relative contraindications to balloon tamponade include an esophageal stricture, recent caustic ingestion, recent esophageal surgery, large hiatal hernia, recent sclerotherapy, congestive heart failure, respiratory failure, cardiac arrhythmias, an unproven variceal source of bleeding, and an improperly trained support staff. Early balloon deflation and tube removal within 24 hours is recommended to prevent pressure necrosis of gastric and esophageal mucosa.

Prevention of Complications. Patients with cirrhosis and admitted for UGIB have a high risk for developing infections that increases with severity of liver disease. The most frequent infections are spontaneous bacterial peritonitis and spontaneous bacteremia (50%), followed by urinary tract infections (25%) and pneumonia (25%). It is recommended that all cirrhotic patients with UGIB receive 7-day course of prophylactic antibiotic therapy.

Prophylaxis of Recurrent Bleeding

The risk of rebleeding after the acute episode can be as high as 30% to 50% within the first day and 60% to 80% within 1 year, thus requiring effective prophylactic measures against rebleeding. Therapies available for prophylaxis of recurrent bleeding include drugs (nonselective beta-blockers and nitrates), EBL, and shunt procedures. According to the guidelines published by the American Association for the Study of Liver Diseases, combination of nonselective beta-blockers plus

EBL is the most optimal approach for secondary prophylaxis. The nonselective beta-blocker should be adjusted to the maximal tolerated dose. Endoscopic band ligation should be repeated every 1 to 2 weeks until obliteration with the first surveillance EGD performed 1 to 3 months after obliteration and then every 6 to 12 months to check for variceal recurrence. Patients who cannot undergo band ligation combination of isosorbide mononitrate and nonselective beta-blocker is recommended. Patients who are Child Class A/B and fail combination therapy of nonselective beta-blockers plus EBL should be considered for TIPS. Finally, patients who are otherwise transplant candidates should be referred to a transplant center for evaluation.

Bleeding from Gastric Varices

The prevalence of gastric varices is 5% to 33% in patients with portal hypertension and is thus less compared to esophageal varices, with a reported incidence of bleeding of about 25% in 2 years. However, bleeding from gastric varices is often more severe. Risk factors for gastric variceal hemorrhage include the size of fundal varices, Child Class (C>B>A), and endoscopic presence of variceal red spots. Compared to EST or EBL, endoscopic variceal obliteration with a tissue adhesive such as N-butyl-cyanoacrylate or isobutyl-2-cyanoacrylate is more effective for acute fundic gastric variceal bleeding. The results include a better rate of controlling the initial hemorrhage as well as lower rebleeding rate. However, in the absence of tissue adhesive agents or unavailability of specialist familiar with the technique, TIPS procedure should be considered first-line therapy. Surgical intervention that includes creation of porto-systemic shunt or gastric devascularization are considered another treatment options.

Portal Hypertensive Gastropathy

Portal hypertensive gastropathy (PHG) are gastric mucosal lesions that, as the name suggests, develop as a result of portal hypertension and generally manifest as chronic gastrointestinal bleeding and chronic anemia. However, these entities may also lead to massive acute gastrointestinal bleeding. They are classically described as a mosaic-like pattern that resembles the skin of a snake, with or without red spots. Endoscopy is the gold standard for diagnosing PHG and is classified according to NIEC as mild when only "mosaic-like pattern" lesions are found or severe when red marks, with or without "mosaic-like pattern" lesions, are present. The incidence of acute upper GI bleeding from PHG varies from 2% to 12%. Acute PHG bleeding can be treated with octreotide or propanolol. Secondary prophylaxis of PHG bleeding with nonselective beta-blockers is recommended.

Selected References

Garcia-Tsao G, Bosch J. Management of varices and variceal hemorrhage in cirrhosis. *N Engl J Med* 2010;362:823–832

Garcia-Pagan JC, Caca K, Bureau C, et al. Early use of TIPS in patients with cirrhosis and variceal bleeding. *N Engl J Med* 2010;362:2370–2379

Chapter 4

Refractory Ascites and Hepatic Hydrothorax

Su Min Cho and Ali Al-Khafaji

Patients with end-stage liver disease (ESLD) can present with several symptoms-related to the presence of fluid in the pleural (hydrothorax) or abdominal cavity (ascites). Hepatic hydrothorax can result from the passage of ascites from the peritoneal to the pleural cavity through small defects in the tendinous portion of the diaphragm. Tense ascites can lead to atelectasis merely from the pressure effect of the fluid on the diaphragm. Even with the presence of minimal amount of ascites, the negative intrathoracic pressure generated during spontaneous inspiration leads to the passage of fluid from the abdomen to the pleural space. Thus, many patients have only mild or no clinically detectable ascites.

Spontaneous bacterial empyema (SBEM) could complicate a simple transudative effusion, and it has some implication on the management of hepatic hydrothorax. SBEM is defined as culture positive pleural fluid or the presence of PMN count greater than 500 cell/μL in the setting of cirrhosis and the absence of parapneumonic effusions.

Chest X-ray is used in diagnosing atelectasis or hepatic hydrothorax. Ultrasound guided thoracentesis should be performed to confirm the diagnosis and to exclude other causes of a pleural effusion. In uncomplicated hepatic hydrothorax, the cell count is low (<500 cells), and the total protein concentration is less than 2.5 g/dL. After performing a thoracenthesis or confirming the lack of a current pleural effusion, a communication between the pleural and the abdominal spaces can be confirmed by the migration of a radioisotope from the abdominal to the pleural cavity after an intra-abdominal injection of the isotope.

Incentive spirometry and other positive pressure breathing maneuvers frequently help in atelectasis. For patients with hepatic hydrothorax, the initial management consists of sodium restriction, diuretics, and thoracentesis. In refractory cases, a transjugular intrahepatic portosystemic shunt (TIPS) or a diaphragmatic repair involving a pleural flap and surgical mesh reinforcement can be an option.

For refractory ascites, in addition to low-sodium-restricted diet, serial large volume paracentesis (intravenous volume replacement), TIPS can be utilized as a treatment option. Liver transplantation is the only definitive therapeutic option.

Selected References

Albillos A, Banares R, Gonzalez M, et al. A meta-analysis of transjugular intrahepatic porto-systemic shunt versus paracentesis forrefractory ascites. *J Hepatol* 2005;43:990–996.

D'Amico G, Luca A, Morabito A, et al. Uncovered transjugular intrahepatic portosystemic shunt for refractory ascites: A metaanalysis. *Gastroenterology* 2005;129:1282–1293.

Gines P, Arroyo V, Vargas V, et al. Paracentesis with intravenous infusion of albumin as compared with peritoneovenous shunting in cirrhosis with refractory ascites. *N Engl J Med* 1991;325:829–835.

Chapter 5

Acute Renal Failure Including Hepatorenal Syndrome

A Maarouf and Ali Al-Khafaji

Definition

Acute kidney injury (AKI) is not uncommon in the setting of liver dysfunction. In general, AKI is defined as a rapid decline in glomerular filtration rate (GFR), leading to accumulation of uremic toxins and derangement in acid-base balance, electrolytes composition, and body fluids homeostasis. Recent efforts to develop a uniform definition of AKI resulted in the establishment of the RIFLE classification (see Table 5.1), which accounts for changes over time in urine output, GFR, and serum creatinine. RIFLE criteria was later modified to describe acute kidney injury in stages, changing the terminology, eliminating the outcome classes (loss and end-stage), and incorporating a rise in creatinine (Cr) in absolute values (see Table 5.2) in addition to the rise in folds used in the original RIFLE classification. The latter change is important when trying to establish the diagnosis of AKI in patients with compensated liver disease, end-stage liver disease (ESLD), or post- orthotopic liver transplantation (OLTx), where the rise in serum Cr could be very subtle but may indicate significant decline in GFR. Creatinine, an end product of muscle catabolism, is the most widely used endogenous filtration marker because of low cost, ease of measurement, and widespread availability. Its serum concentration is affected by low muscle mass, malnutrition, and poor protein intake, factors prevalent in both chronic liver disease and post-OLTx patients. These patients often require fluid resuscitation in the setting of Hepatorenal syndrome (HRS) and massive transfusions of blood products in the peri-operative period, which could dilute the serum concentration of Cr, rendering it a suboptimal marker to detect AKI. In these patients the diagnosis of AKI and the decision to initiate renal replacement therapy often hinges on factors such as the patient's urine output, electrolytes, acid-base, and volume status rather than the rate of increase of their serum BUN and Cr.

Pathophysiology

There are several proposed pathological processes in patients with liver disease that increase their risk of developing renal failure, the most important of which is

Table 5.1 RIFLE Criteria for Acute Renal Failure

Classification	Cr/GFR criteria	Urine Output Criteria
Risk	Increase Serum Cr by 1.5 folds or decrease in GFR >25%	UOP <0.5 mL/kg/hr for 6 hrs
Injury	Increase Serum Cr twofold or decrease GFR >50%	UOP <0.5 mL/kg/hr for 12 hrs
Failure	Increase serum Cr by 3 folds or Cr > 4 mg/dL or acute rise in Cr > 0.5 mg/dL or decrease GFR >75%	UOP <0.3 mL/kg/hr for 24 hrs or anuria for 12 hrs.
Loss	Complete loss of kidney function for >4 weeks	
End-stage	End-stage renal disease for >3 months	

Table 5.2 Acute Kidney Injury Staging (Modified RIFLE)

	Cr criteria	Urine Output Criteria
Stage 1	Increase in serum Cr >0.3 mg/dL or increase in Cr by 1.5- to 2-fold	UOP <0.5 mL/kg/hr for 6 hrs
Stage 2	Increase in serum Cr by more than two- to threefold	UOP <0.5 mL/kg/hr for 12 hrs
Stage 3	Increase in serum Cr by more than threefold or serum Cr >4.0 mg/dL with an acute increase of >0.5 mg/dL or receiving renal replacement therapy	UOP <0.3mL/kg/hr for 24 hrs or anuria for 12 hrs.

disturbances in their circulatory function—namely, decrease in systemic vascular resistance. This is driven by increase in the production of endogenous vasodilators such as nitric oxide, carbon monoxide, and endogenous cannabinoids, which in turn leads to splanchnic arterial vasodilatation. Triggered by portal hypertension, the splanchnic arterial vasodilatation leads to increase in cardiac output to compensate for the reduction in systemic vascular resistance, allowing both arterial pressure and effective circulating volume to remain within normal limits. This increase in cardiac output as a compensating mechanism is overwhelmed by the extent of systemic vascular dilatation in advanced liver disease, so as the disease progresses, underfilling of the arterial circulation ensues. This triggers activation of vasoconstrictor systems such as renin-angiotensin-aldosterone system (RAAS), sympathetic nervous system, and arginine-vasopressin system, which help maintain acceptable arterial pressure and effective circulating arterial volume. Although it maintains arterial pressure and intravascular volume, activation of these vasoconstrictor systems has some untoward effects, including retention of sodium and solute-free water, which may worsen ascites and edema. It also causes intra-renal vasoconstriction with resulting renal hypoperfusion, which may predispose these patients to pre-renal azotemia, acute tubular necrosis (ATN), and HRS. Bacterial translocation has been implicated in the pathogenesis of splanchnic vasodilatation seen in patients with liver disease. It may trigger an inflammatory response leading to the release of proinflammatory cytokines (tumor necrosis factor-alpha and interleukin-6) and vasodilator factors such as nitric oxide, resulting in splanchnic vasodilatation and the associated hemodynamic changes described earlier. A study of selective intestinal decontamination using Norfloxacin revealed partial reversal of the hyperdynamic circulatory state associated with liver cirrhosis, which implicates bacterial translocation in thepathogenesis, although it does not explain the full story. Spontaneous bacterial peritonitis (SBP), like other infectious processes, could be associated with renal failure; however, the severity of renal failure is more pronounced in SBP compared to renal failure associated with other infectious processes. This may result from the severe inflammatory response elicited by the infectious process in the peritoneal cavity, but it is important to realize that a significant amount of renal failure in the setting of SBP is reversible. Given the hemodynamic changes associated with liver failure, renal perfusion is expected to depend on prostaglandin synthesis, and blocking this compensatory mechanism by administering nonsteroidal anti-inflammatory drugs (NSAIDs) may lead to acute renal failure in cirrhotics.

Epidemiology

The incidence of renal failure in liver disease patients is difficult to determine because of the variability of the underlying etiologies of liver disease and whether it is acute versus chronic liver failure. For example, AKI is present in about 75% of patients with acetaminophen overdose and acute liver failure. In a study published in 2002, about 33% of patients who underwent OLTx between 1988 and 1996 had varying degree of renal impairment. This is especially important because the presence of renal dysfunction affects patients' survival while awaiting transplantation and affects both graft and patient survival post-transplantation. Hepatorenal syndrome (see definition below) can affect 18% of cirrhotic patients at 1 year and 35% at 5 years. Independent risk factors for developing HRS include low serum sodium concentration, high serum renin activity, absence of hepatomegaly, low cardiac output, and abnormal resistive index greater than 0.7 on renal dopplers.

Etiology and Clinical Presentation

Simultaneous involvement of both the kidney and the liver is seen in multiple clinical scenarios. For example, some infectious processes could affect both the liver and the kidney at once (Leptospirosis or viral hemorrhagic fevers), sepsis may lead to organ dysfunction in both the liver and kidney resulting from systemic hypoperfusion, and commonly toxic involvement of both organs is seen in cases of acetaminophen overdose. The association between obstructive jaundice and postoperative renal failure is well established in both clinical and animal modules, and some studies have suggested a direct correlation between the level of GFR loss and the degree of hyperbilirubinemia. It is important to approach AKI in patients with liver disease on the basis of pre-, post-, or intrinsic renal failure and routinely investigate common causes of AKI that could occur at increased frequency in patients with advanced liver disease. These patients have systemic and splanchnic vasodilatation that puts them at increased risk for pre-renal azotemia; for example, acute gastrointestinal bleed (varices, gastropathy, ulcer, etc.), diuretics use (treatment of ascites), nausea, vomiting, and diarrhea (resulting from excessive laxative use) may precipitate pre-renal azotemia and lead to ATN. Large volume paracentesis is a particular problem in this patient population, which could induce pre-renal azotemia or type 2 HRS. On the other hand, patients with massive ascites leading to increase in intra-abdominal pressure are at increased risk of AKI resulting from compromise in renal perfusion. Sponatneous bacterial peritonitis and other infections may elicit severe inflammatory response and increased levels of pro-inflammatory cytokines leading to hemodynamic changes that could result in AKI.

It is important to keep in mind that these patients may have an intrinsic kidney disease related to their underlying liver pathology; for example, hepatitis C or B patients may have membranoproliferative (type 1) or membranous glomerulonephritis, respectively. A clue to intrinsic kidney involvement is the presence of proteinuria (>500 mg of protein per day), hematuria (>50 RBCs per high power field), or both.

Also, post-renal etiology should be ruled out by placing Foley's catheter, particularly in elderly men or in patients with hematuria caused by coagulopathy, which increases their risk of obstructing clot and hydronephrosis.

Hepatorenal Syndrome

Hepatorenal syndrome is a functional renal failure in the setting of advanced liver disease characterized by renal vasoconstriction without significant histologic abnormalities. The criteria to diagnose HRS are divided into major and minor and only major criteria are needed for the diagnosis.

Major criteria include excluding other potential etiologies for renal failure, such as the presence of hypotension and shock, SBP, nephrotoxic agents (medications or intravenous contrast), abnormal renal ultrasonography, and parenchymal renal disease (proteinuria > 500 mg/day and/or hematuria > 50 red cells/ high power field). After excluding above etiologies, HRS diagnosis is established by serum creatinine (Cr) level of greater than 1.5 mg/dL, worsening over days or weeks, which does not improve after withdrawal of diuretics, and volume expansion with intravenous albumin at a dose of 1g/kg of body weight (up to 100 g/day) for 2 days.

The minor criteria that supports the diagnosis include urine output (UOP) less than 500 mL/day, urine sodium less than 10 mmol/L, urine osmolality greater than serum osmolality, urine red blood cells less than 50 per hpf, and serum sodium concentration less than 130 mmol/L. Hepatorenal syndrome is divided into two types: HRS type 1 and type 2. Hepatorenal syndrome type 1 is more serious, it frequently follows a precipitating event, survival without treatment is usually in order of weeks, and it is defined as doubling of serum Cr greater than 2.5 mg/dL or a 50% reduction in Cr clearance to less than 20 mL/min in less than 2 weeks. Hepatorenal syndrome type 2 is characterized by slower deterioration of renal function; survival without treatment is usually in order of months, and it mainly presents as diuretic-resistant ascites.

Differential Diagnosis

The combination of liver and renal failure could be seen in cases of shock (hypovolemic, cardiogenic, septic, etc.) and with infections (leptospirosis, brucellosis, tuberculosis, Epstein–Barr virus, hepatistis B and C viruses, HIV, etc.). Some of the drugs that can cause both organs to fail are tetracycline, rifampicin, sulfonamide, phynetoin, allopurinol, methotrexate, and acetaminophen. It can be seen with toxins such as carbon tetrachloride, trichloroetheylene, elemental phosphorus, arsenic, copper, and so forth and amatoxins associated with ingestion of mushrooms of the Amanita genus. Some systemic diseases and malignancies can cause involvement of both organs, such as sarcoidosis, Sjogren's syndrome, systemic lupus erythematosis, amyloidosis, cryoglobulinema, lymphoma, and leukemia. In pregnant women, both liver and kidney failures could be seen with acute fatty liver of pregnancy, HELLP syndrome, and eclampsia.

Management of Renal Failure in Cirrhosis

The care of patients with liver cirrhosis who develop AKI depends on the severity and etiology of their renal failure. In general the management of renal failure is supportive; it involves treatment of the underlying etiology, addressing the complications associated with renal failure, and, in the case of HRS, the use of vasoconstrictors, transjugular intrahepatic portosystemic shunt (TIPS), and ultimately liver transplantation. Cirrhotic patients with significant renal failure are usually managed in intensive care setting as they often have hemodynamic instability and require close hemodynamic monitoring. It is often not easy to assess the optimal amount of volume patients with liver disease require to help restore their intravascular volume, particularly when they have significant peripheral edema. In addition to indications of volume depletion from history, sometimes it is helpful to assess their central venous pressure to guide fluid administration in the absence of cardiac dysfunction or pulmonary hypertension. It is prudent to ensure early assessment and identification of the etiology of renal failure and to address reversible causes. For example, withdrawal of NSAIDs and switching aminoglycosides to less toxic antibiotic regimen could be sufficient to improve renal function. Patients volume status assessment and adequate repletion of their intravascular volume will improve renal failure in cases of pre-renal azotemia from increased gastrointestinal fluid loss caused by nausea, vomiting, and excessive use of lactulose. Discontinuation of all diuretics and using volume expansion will help improve renal function in caused by excessive diuretics use. This will likely prevent progression to acute tubular necrosis. Cirrhotics with gastrointestinal bleeding require, in addition to volume expansion and blood product transfusion, endoscopic intervention to control their variceal bleed. For patients with liver cirrhosis and sepsis caused by SBP, third-generation cephalosporins are the treatment of choice, and patients may benefit from hydrocortisone for relative adrenal insufficiency. Patients with significant ascites undergoing large-volume paracentesis should receive intravenous albumin at a rate of 8 g/L of ascites drained to help alleviate the hemodynamic effects of rapid volume loss on their kidneys perfusion. Patients with liver disease caused by hepatitis C may have cryoglobulinemia and develop rapidly progressive glomerulonephritis resulting from vasculitis, which could be treated with steroids, cytotoxic agents, and plasmapheresis, but the risk of infection and side effects may outweigh the benefits in these patients.

Management of Hepatorenal Syndrome

Several treatment modalities have been utilized in the treatment of HRS, including vasoconstrictor medications, renal vasodilators, TIPS, renal replacement therapy, and molecular adsorbent recirculating system (MARS). Although using renal vasodilators such as prostaglandins, papaverine, phentolamine, and dopamine has not yielded significant benefits, several interventions can prevent and treat HRS, including avoidance of nephrotoxins, adequate volume resuscitation, paracentesis, and vasoconstrictors.

Patients with HRS should be optimally volume resuscitated with intravenous administration of albumin (initially 1 g albumin per kg of body weight, up to a maximum of 100 g, followed by 20–40 g/day) for a maximum of 15 days in combination with terlipressin has been shown to reverse HRS type 1.

In patients with SBP, albumin has been reported to improve systemic hemodynamics and to reduce risk of HRS and death.

Uncontrolled studies demonstrated an improvement in renal function in patients with HRS after paracentesis, likely attributable to increased venous return and cardiac function, and reduced renal venous pressure and intra-renal pressure.

Vasoconstriction of the splanchnic vascular beds is believed to reverse HRS by increasing the effective arterial blood volume, thereby suppressing activation of the renin-angiotensin-aldosterone and the sympathetic nervous systems, therefore reversing compensatory renal vasoconstriction and ultimately increasing renal perfusion.

Midodrine in combination with octreotide and albumin is used in our institution to treat HRS.

Terlipressin, a vasopressin analog, has been shown effective in reversing HRS. An initial pilot study demonstrated that terlipressin improved glomerular filtration rate in patients with HRS compared to placebo.

A retrospective European study has demonstrated survival benefit, particularly as a bridge to liver transplantation. Other studies have confirmed renal function improvement after terlipressin treatment. Albumin infusion in addition to terlipressin therapy led to a complete response in patients with HRS. Vasopressin, norepinephrine, and N-acetylcysteine may play a role in the management of HRS.

The use of nonpharmacological therapy in the treatment of HRS is not well established. The data from an uncontrolled study examining long-term effects of TIPS in nontransplantable HRS patients suggest an improvement in renal function and possible survival advantage. Using TIPS in addition to pharmacotherapy has been investigated in small trials, and data suggest TIPS enhances the improvement of renal function, helps with ascites, and helps in cases where patients relapsed after medical therapy. The balance between risks and benefits of TIPS should be considered, as TIPS carries operative morbidity and mortality.

The use of MARS in the treatment of HRS has been investigated in few small trials. In a prospective controlled trial of 13 patients with liver failure and HRS type 1, eight patients were treated with MARS and medical therapy. In addition, hemodiafiltration (HDF) was used when indicated, and five were treated with HDF and medical treatment alone. The results of the trial suggested improvement in survival, serum sodium level, and bilirubin. Serum Cr level decreased in the study; however, it is difficult to tease out the effects of MARS and HDF on serum Cr level, especially because both treatment modalities have the capacity to clear Cr from blood without true effect on GFR. The latter makes it harder to attribute the decrease in serum Cr seen in the study to true improvement in kidney function, particularly because the slight increase in urine output was not statistically significant.

Using renal replacement therapy (RRT) including intermittent hemodialysis, peritoneal dialysis, and continuous renal replacement therapy (CRRT) has been triggered by their ability to remove toxins implicated in the pathogenesis of hepatic encephalopathy. There are no prospective randomized data to support survival advantage in patients suffering from HRS who are treated with RRT. Moreover, data are lacking to support using CRRT in patients with liver failure who are not candidates for OLTx. Moreover, there are no data comparing RRT with vasoconstrictor administration in patients with HRS, hence, the latter remain the best option we have in the treatment of HRS at this time.

Chronic dialysis in patients with HRS who are not candidates for OLTx has been a controversial topic, primarily because of the increased burden of morbidity and in-hospital stay in these patients when kept alive on dialysis. The decision to place patients with HRS is easy when bridging them for OLTx or when liver failure is acute with expected improvement of liver function; however, in nontransplant candidates, the decision should be made on a case-by-case basis.

Prognosis

In general, renal failure in patients with advanced liver failure carries poor prognosis, with overall survival of about 50% and 20% at 1 month and 6 months, respectively. Survival appears to be particularly worse in patients with HRS, with median survival of 1 month and 6 months in HRS type 1 and 2, respectively. Hence, etiology of renal failure appears to influence survival; in recent prospective studies, both HRS type 1 and model for end-stage liver disease (MELD) score were found to be independent predictors of poor outcome. In contrast, HRS type 2 outcomes were similar to patients with liver failure with renal failure resulting from other etiologies. It is still unclear whether vasoconstrictor therapy improves outcomes in patients with HRS, but patients who respond to such therapy appear to live longer. Ultimately, liver transplantation is the only proven therapy to improve survival in patients with HRS, but we have to keep in mind that severe renal failure is predictive of poor outcome after liver transplantation. It increases the incidence of postoperative sepsis, ICU length of stay, and pre- and postoperative dialysis, and it worsens patients' survival.

Selected References

Davenport A, Ahmad J, Al-Khafaji A, Kellum JA, Genyk YS, & Nadim MK. Medical management of hepatorenal syndrome. *Nephrol Dial Transplant.* 2012;27(1):34–41.

Nadim MK, Kellum JA, Davenport A, Wong F, Davis C, Pannu N, et al. Hepatorenal syndrome: the 8th international consensus conference of the Acute Dialysis Quality Initiative (ADQI) group. *Crit Care.* 2012;16(1):R23.

Chapter 6

Respiratory Failure in Patients With End-Stage Liver Disease

Matthew Cove and Ali Al-Khafaji

Respiratory symptoms are common in chronic liver disease, with 50% to 70% of patients reporting shortness of breath. This reflects the high prevalence of respiratory failure, which, when defined by an arterial pressure of oxygen (PaO_2) of less than 75 mmHg, is present in half of all patients. The causes of respiratory failure are multifactorial, and although much attention is given to portopulmonary hypertension (PPHTN) and the Hepatopulmonary syndrome (HPS), these specific conditions are found in less than 20% of chronic liver failure patients. They are described more fully in the following sections, and although it is important to know about these, the impact of liver disease on respiratory function extends far beyond these two specific conditions.

First, the pathological consequences of chronic liver disease can have a significant impact on pulmonary mechanics. For example, large volume ascites, which frequently develops in liver disease, can result in restricted movement and cephalid displacement of the diaphragm because of the increased intra-abdominal pressure. The overall effect can be a substantial decrease in pulmonary compliance. In addition, ascitic fluid in the peritoneum can leak into the thorax, resulting in the development of a hepatic hydrothorax. Leakage appears to occur through minor defects in the tendious portion of the diaphragm. These defects arise in the tendinous portion of the diaphragm. They are thought to be congenital in origin and enlarge as rising intra-abdominal pressure causing dilatation. Fluid flow from the abdominal to the pleural cavity is further facilitated by negative intrathoracic pressures during inspiration. Hepatic hydrothorax occurs in 5% of patients with end-stage liver disease (ESLD) and can result in compression atelectasis with resultant loss of lung volume available for gas exchange.

As well as alteration of pulmonary mechanics, the presence of liver disease causes notable attenuation of respiratory muscle function. This results from increased turnover of muscle protein and loss of lean body mass, which results in muscle weakness. Abnormal protein metabolism can also contribute to hepatic encephalopathy, which can cause respiratory failure caused by aspiration pneumonitis. Patients with chronic liver disease are also more likely to develop bacterial pneumonitis.

Patients with liver disease are also prone to develop respiratory disorders unrelated to the underlying liver disease. For example, up to 46% of patient with liver cirrhosis are also smokers. It is therefore very common for patients with liver disease to have comorbidities such as emphysema, chronic bronchitis, or obstructive airways disease. Indeed even in the presence of Hepatopulmonary syndrome (see next section), the co-existence of chronic obstructive pulmonary disease is common.

Treatment

Because there are many causes of respiratory failure in the liver patient, treatment is multifaceted and requires complete evaluation of the patient. The contribution of ascites can be immediately improved by changing the patient's position in the bed to reduce the pressure effect on the diaphragm. A more definitive procedure is drainage of the ascites by paracentesis. However, a more effect long-term approach is salt restriction, diuresis and treatment of underlying portal hypertension. The presence of a hepatic hydrothorax or underlying pneumonitis can be assessed by a simple CXR. A hepatic hydrothorax, like ascites, can be treated with diuretics and salt restriction. The use of a chest drain followed by pleurodesis has been advocated in the past; however, it is frequently unsuccessful and may result in increased mortality.

Appropriate care for the patient suffering from chronic liver disease with respiratory failure is therefore a multidisciplinary undertaking typically involving coordinated care provided by internists, gastroenterologists, pulmonologists, physiotherapists, and nutritionalists.

Hepatopulmonary Syndrome

The relationship between the liver and the lungs has intrigued physicians since the late nineteenth century when the combination of liver cirrhosis, clubbing, and hypoxia was first reported. However, it was not until 1977 that the term Hepatopulmonary syndrome (HPS) was established. Hepatopulmonary syndrome is present in 10% to 20% of all patients with chronic liver disease and by definition is a triad of liver disease, a defect in oxygenation and intrapulmonary vascular dilatation.

Much attention has focused on this cause of respiratory failure in liver patients for two reasons. First, its presence denotes a grave prognosis, with a median survival of less than 11 months, compared with more than 40 months in patients with liver cirrhosis alone. Second, in the era of liver transplantation, the observation that HPS improves following transplant makes it presence an important determinant in the prioritization of transplant recipients.

Pathophysiology
Our understanding of the pathophysiology of HPS has developed from the initial observation that some patients who died with liver cirrhosis had marked

dilatation of their pulmonary vasculature. The increased diameter of pulmonary capillaries not only results in increased blood flow but also reduces gas exchange from alveoli, because the distance oxygen has to diffuse to the reach red cells in center of the vessel is increased. When this is combined with the observation that the capillary wall is thickened, it becomes clear that the dilated capillary acts as a shunt. This is because blood can flow through the capillary without being adequately oxygenated, resulting in a significant V-Q mismatch. This is referred to as diffusion-perfusion impairment or alveolar-capillary oxygen disequilibrium.

Diagnosis

Diagnosis of HPS requires the presence of specific clinical features along with confirmatory evidence of pulmonary shunting and intrapulmonary vascular dilatation. Patients with HPS will typically complain of dyspnea; however, as seen in the previous section, this is not specific because there are many reasons that patients with chronic liver disease can develop dyspnea. A characteristic of the dyspnea that is more specific for HPS is platypnea. This is shortness of breath that is worse in the upright position and improves when in the supine position. Platypnea occurs because gravitational effects on blood flow in the upright position cause increased perfusion of the lung bases with consequent worsening of the V-Q mismatch. Additional clinical features that will make the diagnosis of HPS more likely are the presence of spider nevi (cutaneous equivalent of pulmonary vessel dilatation), finger clubbing, and cyanosis.

Laboratory testing, which is necessary to confirm the diagnosis, includes the demonstration of hypoxemia by arterial blood gas analysis. Although many different cutoffs have been used, a PaO_2 less than 70 mmHg in the absence of existing cardiopulmonary disease has a high predictive value for the presence of HPS. In addition, similarly to platypnea, the presence of orthodeoxia is highly specific for HPS in the context of chronic liver disease. By definition, orthodeoxia occurs when there is greater than 5% reduction (or drop >4 mmHg) in PaO_2 when a patient moves from the supine to upright position. Abnormal blood gases should be followed by pulmonary function tests, which will help delineate co-existing pulmonary conditions. Further, the presence of decreased carbon monoxide diffusion capacity is highly sensitive for the presence of HPS. Chest X-ray is typically nonspecific and may be normal even in severe disease.

Dynamic imaging studies are necessary to complete the diagnosis. The simplest and most widely available modality is contrast transthoracic echocardiography, where an intravenous injection of agitated saline is used to demonstrate shunting. In normal circumstances, the microbubbles in the saline will only appear in the right side of the heart because they are trapped and absorbed by the intact pulmonary vasculature. However, in the presence of intracardiac or pulmonary shunts, bubbles can be seen to enter the left side of the heart. These two conditions are distinguished by how quickly the microbubbles appear in the left heart chambers. In the presence of a cardiac shunt, the bubbles transition directly to the left chambers in less than three beats; however, with a pulmonary shunt, it takes three or more beats before the bubbles appear in the left heart chambers. Additional echocardiographic features that would support HPS include right ventricular diastolic dysfunction and a left atrium volume greater than 50 mL.

Technetium macroaggregated albumin perfusion lung scanning can be used to quantify the degree of intrapulmonary shunting. In normal lung, the albumin macroaggregates are trapped by the pulmonary vasculature, but in the presence of intracardiac or intrapulmonary shunts they can pass into the systemic circulation, where they become lodged in other organs. If the uptake in the brain is greater than 6%, then the presence of HPS is likely. However, this method cannot distinguish intracardiac from intrapulmonary shunts.

The gold standard investigation is the demonstration of intrapulmonary vasculature dilatation on pulmonary angiography. However, this is an invasive test, and it is therefore recommended that its use is restricted to patients in whom this form of imaging is likely to change management. Pulmonary angiography demonstrates two patterns of HPS: type 1, in which there is diffuse precapillary and capillary dilatation without arteriovenous fistulas, and type 2, in which focal arteriovenous fistulas are seen. Type 2 represents HPS with a true shunt and should be considered in patients whose PaO2 is less than 200 mmHg on 100% oxygen. It is an important diagnosis to identify because these patients may respond to embolization therapy targeting the arteriovenous shunt. Therefore, it is this group of patients who should go on to receive pulmonary angiography.

Treatment

Despite increased understanding of the role of vasoactive substances in the development of HPS, a successful treatment modality targeting these has remained elusive. Treatment is therefore confined to supportive oxygen therapy, which is helpful in HPS type 1. Increasing the driving force of oxygen across the thickened capillary membrane and into the dilated vessel helps overcome the alveolar-capillary oxygen disequilibrium.

The surprising, but welcome, observation that orthotopic liver transplantation results in reversal of HPS has changed the management of this condition. Indeed it has changed the management of hypoxia in chronic liver disease patients, and hypoxia has changed from being a contraindication to liver transplantation to being a firm indication. The ERS Task Force recommends orthotopic liver transplantation if the PaO2 is 50 to 60 mmHg and consideration, on a case-by-case basis, if the PaO2 is less than 50 mmHg.

Portopulmonary Hypertension

Portopulmonary hypertension was first described in 1951, when surgical exploration of a patient with esophageal abnormalities revealed not only varices but also a large pulmonary artery. Although PPHTN occurs in less than 5% of patients with chronic liver disease, the condition has attracted much interest, not least because of its impact on candidacy for orthotopic liver transplantation.

Portopumonary hypertension is defined as pulmonary hypertension associated with portal hypertension. However, the cause of the portal hypertension may not necessarily be chronic liver disease, and PPHTN has been described in patients with portal hypertension caused by extrahepatic vein occlusion, nonhepatic portal hypertension in SLE, idiopathic portal fibrosis, and primary biliary atresia.

Pathophysiology

The changes seen in PPHTN are similar to those seen in other forms of pulmonary hypertension. These are predominantly abnormalities of vessel wall architecture, which affect the small arteries and arterioles. Typical changes include intimal fibrosis, medial hypertrophy, adventitial proliferation, and fibrinoid necrosis. A characteristic finding is the presence of complex vascular structures composed of endothelial cells called plexiform arteriopathy. Thrombotic lesions and recanalization are also seen; however, these are not thought to be embolic—rather, they appear to develop in situ.

The exact mechanism underlying these changes remains largely unknown, and studies have been hampered by the absence of an effective animal model that recreates PPHTN. Based on current observations, it is quite likely that two events trigger the disease process. First, vessel wall damage occurs as a result of increased blood flow through the pulmonary vasculature caused by increased portal blood return and increased cardiac output. This causes increased vessel wall shear stress, which may trigger a humoral cascade that promotes abnormal remodeling.

Second, there is an imbalance of vasoactive mediators with increased levels of vasoconstrictors and reduced levels of vasodilators. It has been shown that in patients with chronic liver disease, there are increased levels of the potent vasoconstrictor endothelin-1, which is also found in high levels in other forms of pulmonary hypertension. At the same time, the activity of certain vasodilators, such as prostacyclin, is reduced because of reduced synthesis. When combined, these two events result is disregulation of the pulmonary vasculature.

Diagnosis

The diagnosis of PPHTN is largely made by demonstrating the presence of pulmonary hypertension in a patient with portal hypertension. By definition pulmonary hypertension is a mean pulmonary artery pressure (PAP) equal to or greater than 25 mmHg with a pulmonary artery occlusion pressure less than 15 mmHg. Symptoms associated with PPHTN are variable and range from mild dyspnea on exertion to chest pain and syncope. Unlike HPS, patients with PPHTN tend to develop orthopnea rather than platypnea.

Clinical features seen in PPHTN are related to worsening right heart function and typically do not manifest until advanced disease is present. This is partly because early features such as peripheral edema and ascites are difficult to distinguish from the underlying liver disease itself. Clinical findings consistent with advanced right heart failure include an elevated jugular venous pressure, widened splitting of the second heart sound with a prominent P2, right ventricular heave, and a pulsatile liver. In these patients, arterial blood gases will typically demonstrate mild hypoxia, and an EKG will demonstrate findings consistent with right ventricular strain (R-wave in V1, right bundle branch block, and rightward axis deviation). Chest X ray (CXR) findings are nonspecific, and pulmonary function tests are only helpful for exclusion of alternative causes of respiratory insufficiency.

Diagnosis is confirmed by measuring the PAP, and this routinely is performed indirectly using transthoracic echocardiography. Pulmonary artery systolic pressure can be estimated by measuring the velocity of the tricuspid regurgitant jet. By using the modified Bernoulli equation, the velocity of the regurgitant can be used to determine the trans-tricuspid pressure gradient during systole. By adding the estimated right atrial pressure to this value, the systolic right ventricular pressure—and hence pulmonary artery pressure—can be determined. Using a similar calculation, the pulmonary diastolic pressure and mean pulmonary artery pressure can be calculated from the velocity of the regurgitant jet across the pulmonary valve in diastole. These measurements can be difficult to obtain in some patients and are prone to significant interoperator variation. Therefore, it is recommended that a right heart catheter is performed in any patient who has an estimated pulmonary artery systolic pressure greater than 50 mmHg so that the pressures can be measured directly.

Treatment

Unlike HPS, untreated persistent PPHTN is a contraindication to transplant because it is associated with high perioperative mortality. Patients with a mean PAP greater than 50 mmHg have a 100% risk of mortality post-transplant, and patients with a mean PAP 35 to 50 mmHg have a 50% risk of mortality. However, a mean PAP less than 35 mmHg is not a contraindication for transplant surgery, and if the PPHTN can be medically managed to achieve a mean PAP less than 35 mmHg, the pulmonary vasculature may normalize following transplant, albeit after many months or years. The goal of treatment for POPH is therefore to control the mean PAP to allow orthotopic liver transplantation.

Medical options for management of POPH are similar to those used in other forms of pulmonary hypertension. Supportive therapy with oxygen to maintain hemoglobin saturations greater than 90% will reduce any hypoxia-induced pulmonary vasoconstriction. Gentle diuretic therapy will help reverse the volume overload state in which these patients typically exist; however, it does happen at the cost of cardiac output, when there is significant right heart failure present.

The use of vasodilation medications require careful consideration in PPHTN patients. In most patients with pulmonary hypertension, calcium channels have proven effective. However, in patients with PPHTN, this class of medication may increase the hepatic venous pressure gradient and increase the risk of variceal hemorrhage. The most studied vasodilators for the treatment of PPHTN are prostanoids and phosphodiesterase-5 inhibitors. Epoprostenol is a prostenoid that reduces the mean PAP in patients with PPHTN by activating endothelial prostacyclin receptors, which causes both vasodilation and reduced smooth muscle proliferation. Its use is complicated by the fact that it can only be given through a centrally placed intravenous catheter. Although it is unclear whether prostanoids alone improve mortality, when combined with orthotopic liver transplantation, they do result in improved survival. Sildenafil is a phosphodiesterase-5 inhibitor that has shown promise in PPHTN. It works by blocking degradation of the second messenger of nitric oxide (cyclic guanasine monophosphate), thereby potentiating its vasodilatory effects. The advantage of sildenafil over epoprostenol is that it can be taken orally. A suitable approach to treatment of PPHTN would therefore involve supportive oxygen therapy and sildenafil, and if these measures fail to achieve a mean PAP less than 35 mmHg, then the addition of epoprostenol prior to consideration for orthotopic liver transplantion should be considered.

Difference Between Portopulmonary Hypertension and Hepatopulmonary Syndrome

	Portopulmonary Hypertension	Hepatopulmonary Syndrome
Presence of portal hypertension	Yes	Yes
Cause	Pulmonary vascular vasoconstriction Endothelial smooth muscle proliferation In situ thrombosis and fibrosis Remodeling of arterial wall	Right-to-left shunt Pulmonary vascular dilation
Presence of right heart failure	Happen at late stage	None present
Presence of pulmonary hypertension	Yes	No
Diagnosis	Excertional dyspnea Fatigue Syncope and chest pain in severe cases High mean pulmonary artery pressure High pulmonary vascular resistance	Platypnea Orthodeoxia Normal pulmonary hemodynamics Right-to-left shunt on TTE Decrease carbon monoxide diffusion capacity Intrapulmonary vascular dilation on pulmonary angiogram

	Portopulmonary Hypertension	Hepatopulmonary Syndrome
Treatment	Vasodilators	Oxygen
	Liver transplant	Liver transplant
		Embolization of shunt in selected cases
Resolution post-liver transplant	Yes but may take months to years	Yes

Adopted from Al-Khafaji A & Huang DT. Critical care management of patients with end-stage liver disease. *Crit Care Med.* 2011;39(5):1157–1166.

Selected Reference

Krowka MJ, Plevak DJ, Findlay JY, et al. Pulmonary hemodynamics and perioperative cardiopulmonary-related mortality in patients with portopulmonary hypertension undergoing liver transplantation. *Liver Transpl* 2000;6:443–450.

Chapter 7

Malnutrition in Chronic Liver Disease

Rebecca Gooch, Ali Al-Khafaji, and Stephen O'Keefe

The liver plays a pivotal role in integrating the biochemical pathways that regulate carbohydrate, fat, protein, and vitamin metabolism, and thus malnutrition becomes a common and serious complication of liver disease.

Malnutrition is as serious a complication as ascites, esophageal varices, and hepatic encephalopathy and has been shown to be present up to 25% of the time in patients with even mild liver disease. The significance of malnutrition is considerable. Malnourished cirrhotic patients have a significant increase in morbidity and morality, and it has been shown that early intervention in addressing nutritional needs can prolong life expectancy, improve quality of life, and decrease complications as well as prepare them for a more successful liver transplantation.

Causes of Malnutrition

Diminished Intake

Anorexia
Intestinal malabsorption
Iatrogenic etiologies

Hypermetabolic State

Inadequate Synthesis or Absorption of Micro- and Macronutrients
Diminished nutrient intake is a common cause of malnutrition in chronic liver disease and is largely the result of decreased appetite and early satiety. Decreased appetite is the result of a combination of factors, including increased circulating levels of the cytokines—specifically tumor necrosis factor-alpha (TNF-α), interleukin (IL)-1b and IL-6, and alcohol-induced anorexia. Zinc deficiency, which is the result of decreased absorption and the use of diuretics leading to urinary zinc excretion, also contributes to the loss of appetite, as does hyperglycemia and unpalatable diets of sodium and protein restriction.

Impaired gastric compliance as well as decreased stomach expansion resulting from ascites are often contributory factors to early satiety. It has been shown that large volume paracentesis increases fasting gastric volumes, which was associated with a significant increase in the tolerated volumes during caloric intake over a 3-day period.

Intestinal malabsorption also contributes to decreased nutrient intake. Portal hypertension impairs digestion, and cholestatic liver disease decreases absorption—especially of fat-soluble vitamins (ADEK). In addition, bacterial overgrowth, coexistent small bowel disease, pancreatic insufficiency, mucosal congestion, and villus atrophy also contribute to the impaired absorption and utilization of nutrients. The causes of malnutrition are multifactorial, and a common contributing factor is the tendency of physicians to prescribe a low-protein diet to prevent hepatic encephalopathy. In addition, the frequent hospitalizations with procedures and examinations can disregulate meals and result in the prolonged fasting of patients.

Hypermetabolic State

Cirrhotic patients are often found to have disturbances in metabolic rate. It has been shown that approximately 34% of cirrhotics are hypermetabolic with resting energy expenditure 120% of normal. This results from a variety of factors, one of which is the hyperdynamic circulatory changes that occur with cirrhosis. These changes include systemic vasodilatation and expanded intravascular blood volume, which lead to more work for the heart, requiring an increase in the use of macro- and micronutrients. Hypermetabolism is also thought to be related to the pro-inflammatory and anti-inflammatory cytokine levels that are elevated in the cirrhotic patient. Decreased glycogen stores can also precipitate hypoglycemia and induce gluconeogenesis, with further proteolysis and catabolism. Finally, the multiple complications that can occur in a cirrhotic patient—spontaneous bacterial peritonitis, hepatic encephalopathy, and bleeding—can all lead to a stressed physiologic state and increased energy expenditure driving a patient into catabolism. This can often lead to a marked decrease in the patient's nutritional state.

Inadequate Synthesis or Absorption of Nutrients

The cirrhotic liver and its damaged hepatocytes have a decreased hepatic glycogen reserve, and it has been noted that when cirrhotic patients are fasted overnight, their body mobilizes amino acids from skeletal muscle to initiate gluconeogenesis and provide the body with its required glucose. To illustrate just how damaged the hepatic cells are in cirrhosis, the switch to gluconeogenesis from amino acids is observed in healthy individuals after 3 days of fasting.

As mentioned previously, fat-soluble vitamin malabsorption largely results from the cholestasis and portal hypertensive enteropathy. Osteoporosis can result from the combined effect of decreased Vitamin D and calcium, and Vitamin K deficiency can worsen coagulopathy. Vitamin A is often deficient, as is folate, riboflavin, nicotinamide, pantothenic acid, pyroxidine, Vitamin B12, and thiamine.

Minerals such as Zinc, magnesium sodium, and phosphate are also often deficient. Zinc deficiency as mentioned above can alter appetite and taste, but it also will impair wound healing, protein metabolism, and the immune system.

Protein is also just simply lost in the cirrhotic patient by the occult or overt bleeding from esophageal and gastric varices, as well as from the incompetent intestinal lumen with protein losing enteropathy.

Protein deficiency from whatever etiology results in the imbalance of branched-chain amino acids (BCAAs) (leucine, isoleucine, and valine) and aromatic amino acids (phenylalanine, methionine, and tyrosine). The expected ratio should be 3:5:1; however, this ratio falls to 1:1 in patients with end-stage liver disease (ESLD), allowing increased cerebral uptake of false neurotransmitters, which may affect neurocognitive function. Very simply, the brain's uptake of tryptophan is increased in patients with hepatic encephalopathy. Branched-chain amino acids and tryptophan compete for the same amino acid transporter on the blood–brain barrier, and when the ratio of BCAAs to tryptophan is decreased, more tryptophan is allowed to pass into the brain circulation, contributing to hepatic encephalopathy.

Assessment of Malnutrition

To assess the degree of malnutrition in the patient with liver disease, a variety of factors must be evaluated. A thorough medical history, physical examination, and dietary history must be obtained. Topics that should specifically be addressed are the degree of anorexia, early satiety, weight changes, taste abnormalities, and the presence of chronic diarrhea. These topics make up the Subjective Global Assessment, which is currently the recommended practical bedside method for assessing undernourished patients by the European Society for Clinical Nutrition and Metabolism (ESPEN). The European Society for Clinical Nutrition and Metabolism also recommends the use of simple anthropometric parameters in evaluating malnutrition. These parameters are not affected by the presence of ascites and peripheral edema, and include mid-arm muscle circumference and triceps skin-fold thickness. Laboratory tests of interest include a complete blood count to assess for anemia, bilirubin and albumin levels, and prothrombin time to assess synthetic liver function. These tests will reflect liver dysfunction and portal hypertension but do not necessarily correlate to body cell mass. Body cell mass represents the active metabolic body compartment and is responsible for basal energy expenditure. Sensitive markers of body cell mass depletion have shown to be mid-arm muscle circumference and handgrip strength measurements. Additional methods of body mass composition include bioelectrical impedance analysis, which evaluates the body electrical conductivity and resistance and has been used to determine the lean body mass and fat in patients with liver disease. It is an inexpensive test, but the measurement may be inaccurate because of the presence of edema in most patients with ESLD.

Dual-energy X-ray absorptiometry is another test that can be used to measure total body bone, mineral, fat, and fat-free mass, but it also may be inaccurate in patients with fluid retention.

Repleting the Nutritional Deficit

Nutritional health is an important goal for patients with ESLD. Weight should be maintained through a diet rich in macro- and micronutrients. It is recommended that patients with liver cirrhosis receive 35 to 40 kcal/kg per day, with a protein intake up to 1.6 g/kg per day as a continuous infusion in severe cases to prevent starvation hypoglycemia. A normal diet without restriction should be the standard in patients with compensated liver disease. Those with uncompensated liver disease may need a more specific dietary regimen, including supplementary meals and no protein restriction.

Around 40% to 50% of all patients with ESLD have diabetes mellitus. The cause of this is multifactorial, with the most common being insulin resistance. Other etiologies include pancreatic injury resulting from alcohol toxicity, diminished glycogen storage capacity of the liver, and the impaired glucose uptake from the skeletal muscles. Even so, carbohydrate intake should not be restricted in patients with ESLD. Hypoglycemia is common and serious, leading to brain injury resulting from the decreased synthetic function of hepatocytes and increased insulin levels. Patients with ESLD benefit the most from multiple small meals through the day, and an evening snack prior to sleep is specifically advised to avoid the overnight fasting state that occurs in cirrhotic patients.

The cirrhotic liver also loses the ability to synthesize very low-density lipoprotein (VLDL). Therefore, it cannot excrete fat from the liver. As it gets absorbed and transported to the liver through the portal system, the result is an increased uptake and storage in the hepatocytes, further stressing these already damaged cells. Enteral feeding is recommended when a patient's oral intake is not meeting daily caloric requirement. Tube feeding is advised even if the patient has esophageal varices or bleeding varices. Tube feed formula should be selected based on the individual needs of the patient. Concentrated high-energy, high-protein formulas are advised in patients with ascites. Patients who develop hepatic encephalopathy with enteral feeding are candidates for BCAA formulations. A BCAA-enriched, aromatic amino acid depleted formula is theoretically the best formula for patients with hepatic failure, as aromatic amino acids can only be removed by the liver whereas BCAA are avidly metabolized by skeletal muscle as well. The European Society for Clinical Nutrition and Metabolism has recommended the administration of BCAA for this reason.

As described earlier, BCAAs are an important factor in hepatic encephalopathy but also have a role in energy metabolism. In addition to being a substrate for protein synthesis, they also help regulate protein synthesis and keep skeletal muscles intact. Because of this, BCAAs have been postulated to help cirrhotic patients shift from a catabolic to an anabolic state and have been looked at as an oral supplement for patients with ESLD.

Multiple studies have investigated the utility in BCAA supplementation, which is most beneficial if given as the late evening snack. It has been shown to prevent the overnight fast that occurs in cirrhotics and to increase hepatic albumin synthesis. Daytime administration showed that the BCAA was used primarily for energy and not for albumin synthesis and, therefore, had less benefit. Vitamins and minerals should be supplemented to prevent deficiency.

Parental nutrition may be necessary in certain cases such as the lack of functional gut.

SCCM/ASPEN Kilocalorie and Protein Recommendations Based on BMI.			
BMI	Weight for Computation	Kilocalories (per kg)	Protein** (g/kg)
<30	Actual	25	1.5
30–34.9	Ideal	22	2.0
35–39.9	Ideal	22	2.0
≥40	Ideal	22	2.5
Presence of significant ascites or edema*	Ideal or Dry Wt (If Known)	25	1.5

*BMI will not be accurate in patient with edema/ascites.

**Protein requirements may need to be adjusted in patients with decompensated liver disease and renal failure without dialysis.

Based on BMI.

Selected Reference

O'Keefe SJD, El-Zayadi AR, Carraher TE, Davis M, & Williams R. Malnutrition and immuno-incompetence in patients with liver disease. *Lancet* 1980;2(8195 pt1):615–617.

Section 2

Transplantation

Chapter 8

General Principle of Immunosuppression

Deanna Blisard

Post-transplant immunosuppression almost always includes a combination of drugs and approaches based on a patient's individual situation, organ transplanted, and current developments in the field. Depending on these factors, approaches could include:

- Induction immunosuppression. This approach includes all medications given in the initial days after transplantation in intensified doses for the purpose of preventing acute rejection. They are not used long-term for immunosuppressive maintenance. Associated medications can include methylprednisolone, Atgam, thymoglobulin, OKT3, basiliximab (Simulect), or daclizumab (Zenapax).
- Maintenance immunosuppression. Maintenance includes all immunosuppressive medications given before, during, or after transplant with the intention to maintain them long term. This type of immunosuppression does not include medications given for rejection episodes or induction. These include prednisone, cyclosporine, tacrolimus, mycophenolate mofetil, azathioprine, and rapamycin.
- Anti-rejection immunosuppression. This approach includes all immunosuppressive medications given for the purpose of treating an acute rejection episode. Associated medications can include methylprednisolone, Atgam, OKT3, thymoglobulin, basiliximab, daclizumab, or campath.

There are numerous protocols and combinations available depending on the organ transplanted, rejection history, and transplant center. A discussion involving all of these combinations are beyond the scope of this chapter.

Azathioprine

Azathioprine and steroids were the backbone of immunosuppression from the early 1960s up to the early 1980s, when cyclosporine became available. Azathioprine has largely been replaced with the introduction of mycophenolate mofetil and sirolimus, both of which are antiproliferative agents. Its main mechanism of action is the inhibition of DNA and RNA synthesis by preventing interconversion among purine synthesis precursors. It also suppresses de novo purine synthesis. Azathioprine blocks lymphocyte proliferation in vitro and production of interleukin (IL)-2 (which is an important aspect of its antiproliferative activity).

Side Effects

The major side effect of azathioprine is bone marrow aplasia, with leukopenia being the primary line affected. Regular leukocyte monitoring is especially important for patients on azathioprine. Megaloblastic anemia can also be present. Other side effects attributed to azathioprine use are hepatotoxicity (rare, and other causes should be actively sought out) and hair loss.

Steroids

Steroid use increased in patients suffering from acute rejection while on azathioprine, but steroids were added as maintenance immunosuppression by Dr Thomas Starzl to prevent rejection. Dosing of steroids during this time was large, with a gradual reduction to maintenance levels over 6 to 12 months. In the 1970s, several randomized trials and observational studies led to low-dose steroid regimens. Although steroids will continue to have a role in preventing and treating rejection, with the introduction of powerful new agents, steroid-sparing protocols are being looked at.

Mechanism of Action

The common formulation of steroids used is either prednisone or prednisolone. Steroids have a complex and not fully understood mechanism of action, with anti-inflammatory and immunosuppressive properties. In the event of acute rejection, the anti-inflammatory activity is what probably produces the immediate response. In prophylaxis, the immunosuppressive properties predominate.

Steroids have an in vitro effect on T-cell proliferation, blocking IL-2 production. Other actions augment steroids' immunosuppressive activity, such as preventing induction of IL-1 and IL-6. The anti-inflammatory effect may be mediated by monocyte migration inhibition to the areas of inflammation. The same activity affects wound healing.

Treatment of Acute Rejection

High-dose steroids are the first-line therapy for an acute rejection. Early approaches involved either increasing the oral dose to very high levels (200 mg/day for 3 days), with a rapid decrease over 10 days to the previous dosage or boluses of IV methylprednisolone (0.5–1 g/day for 3–5 days).

Side Effects

There are numerous side effects of maintenance steroid therapy. However, with the steroid-sparing and low-dose steroid protocols in use now, there appears to be decreased side effects.

o Cushingoid facies—used to be hallmark of patients on steroids, including moon face, buffalo hump, acne, and obese torso. This is less frequent with lower doses.
o Wound healing—this is a result of the anti-inflammatory effect; it is less of an issue, but surgical clips and sutures are left in the transplant patient for 2 to 3 weeks.
o Diabetes—glycosuria and insulin-/non-insulin-dependent diabetes are common. This is in part related to steroid use. It is more commonly seen when steroids are used simultaneously with calcineurin inhibitors.
o Hyperlipidemia—cyclosporine also increases the lipid profile. It has been shown that withdrawal of steroids improves the lipid profile.
o Bone disease—is common, especially in post-menopausal women. Avascular necrosis of the femur was a common occurrence (10%–15% within 2 years of transplantation). The incidence is decreasing with low-dose protocols.
o Obesity—steroids increase both appetite and salt and water retention.
o Hypertension—found to be partly related to steroid use, as steroid withdrawal improves the blood pressure.
o Psychiatric disturbances—can be seen in patients on steroids in two ways: high-dose steroids presenting with significant mood changes and during withdrawal of steroids presenting with depression.
o Cataracts—steroid-related cataracts can occur in up to 25% after renal transplantation.

Cyclosporine

Cyclosporine was isolated from two strains of imperfect fungi (*Cylindrocarpon lucidium booth* and *trichoderma polysporum Rifai*) from soil samples as an antifungal agent. Clinical trials in renal transplant began in Cambridge in 1978. Cyclosporine became commercially available for transplantation in the 1980s.

Mechanism of Action

Cyclosporine's predominant action is directed against CD4 (T-helper) lymphocytes. It prevents production of lymphokines, especially IL-2, which inhibits the further proliferation of CD4+ T cells and the generation of cytotoxic T cells from the cytotoxic T-cell precursor.

Cyclosporine binds within the cytosol to cyclophilin (cis-trans-peptidyl-polyl isomerase) that plays a role in the folding of proteins and peptides. Most of the drug binds to cyclophilin A. The complex made up of cyclosporine and cyclophilin is the immunosuppressive molecule. Cyclosporine is actually a prodrug. This complex binds to a calcium- and calmodulin-dependent phosphatase (calcineurin). Calcineurin is crucial in the transduction of calcium-dependent signals leading to activation of IL-2.

Although the decreased IL-2 production and IL-2 receptor expression with resultant reduction of T-cell activation is the main path of action, others are thought to exist.

Dosing

Cyclosporine can be combined with steroids or used as monotherapy. In the United States, the tendency has been to use high-dose steroids. Many transplant patients can be managed without steroids or weaned early. In the past, monotherapy was achieved with high doses of cyclosporine (17.5 mg/kg/day). Many of the side effects of cyclosporine are dose related and can be attributed to these high doses. With further experience, doses were able to be decreased based on trough levels; levels of 200 to 400 ng/mL are targeted in the early postoperative period and 100 to 200 ng/mL after. Traditional monitoring looks at the trough levels (Co levels). The relation between the Co level and nephrotoxicity is nonlinear and correlates poorly with rejection rates.

Drug Interactions

Cyclosporine is metabolized almost entirely in the liver by the cytochrome P450 system. Most of the drug is excreted in bile. Inducers of the P450 system will decrease cyclosporine levels. Some of the more common medications include nafcillin, octreotide, phenytoin, and rifampicin. Inhibitors of P450 will increase cyclosporine levels and include allopurinol, amiodarone, diltiazem, fluconizole, macrolides, and metoclopramide. Synergistic effects are seen with amphotericin B, ciprofloxacin, gentamycin, rapamycin, tacrolimus, bactrim, and vancomycin. There are also dietary considerations—taking cyclosporine with grapefruit juice will increase the cyclosporine level by up to 37%, whereas vitamins C and E will decrease the level.

Side Effects

The most concerning side effect related to cyclosporine is nephrotoxicity. It exerts its toxic effect on three stages: immediately after transplant (usually related with ischemia). Acute nephrotoxicity is usually greater than 2 to 3 weeks and presents with decreased renal function and usually a high cyclosporine trough. It is important to distinguish nephrotoxicity because of cyclosporine from acute cellular rejection, as the treatments are different. A renal biopsy is usually needed to make the distinction. Chronic toxicity presents with a slow steady deterioration of renal function. Histology may reveal severe interstitial fibrosis.

Other side effects of cyclosporine include:

- Hepatotoxicity—usually presents with temporarily increased liver function tests

- Neoplastic—linked to promotion of tumor angiogenesis by vascular endothelial growth factor dependent mechanism
- Dermatologic—skin is the principle site of accumulation, and includes gum hypertrophy and hypertrichosis
- Metabolic—hyperkalemia, which is reversible with a decrease in the dose. The mechanism is unclear and may be related to a decrease in serum aldosterone or primary tubular defect. It also includes an increase in urate and decreased magnesium with increased cyclosporine levels. Glycosuria and hyperglycemia (likely resulting from inhibition of insulin secretion and glucose intolerance) are also seen.
- Neurologic—tremor, convulsions, parasthesias, mania, and depression
- Cardiovascular—hypertension and hyperlipidemia
- Hematologic—ABO autoimmune hemolytic anemia (O kidney into A or B recipient, although more commonly seen in liver transplantation)
- Antiviral—cyclosporine may be anti-HIV and anti-HCV by binding to cyclophilin A. Cyclophilin A is involved in maturation and replication of HIV-1 and HCV cyclophilin B.

Tacrolimus

Tacrolimus shows superior clinical outcomes in liver and kidney transplants. It was isolated in 1984 from *Streptomyces tsukubaensis* (a soil organism). The initial clinical trial as the primary immunosuppression in liver transplantation was performed in 1990 at the University of Pittsburgh Medical Center.

Mechanism of Action

Tacrolimus binds to FK BP-12, an intracellular protein. The complex of tacrolimus (FK BP-12, calcium, calmodulin, and calcineurin) inhibits the phosphatase activity of calcineurin. This complex prevents dephosphorylation and translocation of nuclear factor of activated T cells, which initiates gene transcription for formation of IL-2. Tacrolimus is 10 to 100 times more potent than cyclosporine. It also inhibits NO synthetase activation and apoptosis and potentiates steroid action in apoptosis.

Tacrolimus is metabolized by the cytochrome P40 (CYP) 3A4 isoenzyme. Tacrolimus concentrations are increased by calcium channel blockers, imidazole antifungals, macrolide antibiotics, and prokinetics. Anticonvulsants and rifampicin, as well as others, decrease its concentration.

Side Effects

The side effect profile is very similar to cyclosporine. Concomitant use of both calcineurin inhibitors is contraindicated because of acute and chronic nephrotoxicity. Nephrotoxicity is dose related and responds to dosage decrease.

Other side effects include:
- Hyperlipidemia, although there is a better lipid profile versus cyclosporine-based regimens.
- Hypertension is also common with the calcineurin inhibitors.
- Post-transplant diabetes mellitus. The incidence is reported in a meta-analysis as 9.8% versus 2.7% for tacrolimus versus cyclosporine.
- Alopecia
- Tremor
- Headache
- Insomnia
- Vomiting
- Diarrhea
- Hypomagnesiumia (more than cyclosporine).

Mycophenolate Mofetil

Mycophenolate mofetil (MMF) is a fermentation product from *Penicillium brevi compactum* and related fungi. Its primary action is to inhibit nucleic acid synthesis.

Mechanism of Action
Mycophenolate acid (MPA) causes a rapid reversible noncompetitive inhibition of IMDPH, which is the rate-limiting enzyme in de novo synthesis of guanine. It stops new DNA synthesis in proliferating cells at G1/S interface, with GTP levels decreased to 10% of those in unstimulated T cells.

Side Effects
In initial clinical trials, MMF lacks the nephrotoxicity, neurotoxicity, and hepatotoxicity of the calcineurin inhibitors. It does have modest myelotoxicity and gastrointestinal side effects.

The gastrointestinal side effects can include diarrhea, indigestion with nausea, vomiting, pain, and reflux. Diarrhea is the most common complaint. Colonic biopsies show apoptosis of intestinal gland epithelial cells. MMF-induced diarrhea may decrease cyclosporine concentrations but markedly increase tacrolimus concentrations.

The myelosuppression from MMF must be distinguished from poor allograft function, iron deficiency, and viral infections. Leukopenia is the common form of myelosuppression and may be associated with markedly abnormal neutrophil morphology. It is also associated with stomatitis.

When MMF is compared to azathioprine, there is an increased incidence and severity of tissue-invasive CMV, herpes, zoster, and BK virus. There is a significant increase in HCV viremia when used with cyclosporine. A large prospective observational cohort study failed to show an increased risk of lymphoma or malignancy associated with MMF versus other immunosuppression agents. However, MMF does not slow neoplastic cell division like sirolimus, and conversion from MMF to sirolimus is likely indicated when neoplasm present.

Cough, dyspnea, and increased sputum production likely represents a bronchiectasis condition. Conversion to another agent resolves symptoms.

Sirolimus or Rapamune (mTOR inhibitor)

This agent impairs T-cell proliferation by inhibiting mammalian target of Rapamycin (mTOR). It is a fermentation product of *Streptomyces hygroscopicus*, which is taken from Easter Island soil (Rapa Nui). It was first isolated for use as an antifungal agent but found to inhibit tumor cell growth and decrease lymphocyte proliferation.

Mechanism of Action

Sirolimus enters cells and binds to one of the family of immunophilins called FK506-binding protein. Sirolimus–FKBP12 complexes with mTOR 55, a serine-threonine kinase that is the scaffold for binding of other proteins, and a key component of cell cycle regulatory signaling pathway. The result is cell cycle arrest in late G1 phase. Sirolimus also has a direct inhibitory effect on dendritic cells, including apoptosis through interaction with growth factor signaling. Metabolism is by the cytochrome P450 3A (CYP3A4 and CYP3A5) system.

There are interactions with other immunosuppression medications of which one should be aware. Cyclosporine can increase sirolimus with a reciprocal increase in cyclosporine concentrations. It decreases the exposure to tacrolimus when co-administered. Antimicrobials and statins also alter sirolimus concentrations. It also increases exposure to MMF.

Side Effects

A significant side effect of sirolimus is hyperlipidemia. Two-thirds of patients can develop increased triglycerides, with half developing hypercholesterolemia. Lipids are implicated in the development of cardiovascular disease and the genesis of chronic rejection. It has been shown to prevent accelerated vascular disease in cholesterol-fed, apolipoprotein-E-deficient mice despite high cholesterol levels.

Other significant side effects include:
- Pneumonitis characterized by progressive dyspnea, dry cough, fatigue, fever, and can lead to pulmonary failure.
- Poor wound healing, implicated in poor airway anastamotic healing in lung transplants
- Hematological side effects include anemia, thrombocytopenia, and leukopenia
- May increase hepatic artery thrombosis when used with cyclosporine.
- Mucositis is expressed as gingival or buccal mucosa ulcerations.

- The rashes are an inflammatory acneiform eruption or dermatitis like rash mostly on hands and fingers.
- Hemolytic uremic syndrome (thrombotic microangiopathy)
- Angioedema of eyelid and tongue
- Hypokalemia
- Hypophosphatemia

Antibodies

Polyclonal Antibodies

Polyclonal antibodies include antithymocyte globulin from rabbit (Thymoglobulin) and horse (Atgam). These antibodies have been used to achieve immunosuppression since the 1960s. They are used in induction and rescue therapies. There is no single mechanism of action.

In the 1960s to 1970s, polyclonal antibodies were used to increase or augment the effects of steroids and azathioprine to decrease the incidence of acute cellular rejection. Usually a 2- to 3-week course of the polyclonal antibody would delay onset of rejection and decrease the use of high-dose steroids early. Since the discovery and use of cyclosporine, polyclonal antibody use has fallen off because of an increased risk of infection and malignancy.

Polyclonal antibodies are used in steroid-resistant acute cellular rejection. Most ACR in the cyclosporine or tacrolimus era respond to high-steroid bolus, with the polyclonal antibodies used as second-line treatment. Thymoglobulin is better than Atgam in rescue scenarios.

The administration of thymoglobulin needs to be via a large-caliber central vein to avoid thrombophlebitis. The usual dose is 1.5 mg/kg/dose for a total of 7.5 to 10mg/kg. Each dose is given over 4 to 6 hours. The acute side effects are related to a transient cytokine release and include fevers and chills. Side effects are usually effectively treated by pre-medicating with steroids, an antipyretic, and an antihistamine. Longer-term side effects of polyclonal antibodies are associated with an increased reactivation and development of viral diseases such as cytomegalovirus (CMV), HSV, Epstein–Barre virus (EBV), and varicella.

Leukopenia and thrombocytopenia are countered by dose adjustment of thymoglobulin. Fever, urticaria, rash, and headache are also common and related to the release of pyrogenic cytokines tumor necrosis factor (TNF)-gamma, IL-1, and IL-6. Less frequently pulmonary edema and severe hypertension or hypotension can lead to death.

Monoclonal Antibodies

Monoclonal antibodies (MAbs) differ from polyclonal preparations in that all antibody molecules are derived from a single genetic template and are identical. The most commonly used monoclonal antibody is muromonab (OKT3), a murine-anti CD3 drug. OKT3 is an IgG2a mouse antibody that binds to the epsilon component of human CD3 (expressed on all T cells). Once bound, the antibody mediates complement-dependent cell lysis and ADCC, thereby rapidly clearing T cells from the circulation.

Induction with OKT3 cannot prevent ACR beyond the actual infusion without maintenance immunosuppression. It is mostly useful in sensitized patients and delayed graft function (DGF) by helping to delay use of calcineurin inhibitors and avoiding nephrotoxicity. Its primary use is in biopsy-proven, steroid-resistant ACR. It shows a sustained reversal of rejection in 80% of cases.

The side effects of OKT3 include fever, nausea/vomiting, rigors, and general malaise, which are similar to severe flu-like symptoms. It increases vascular permeability and may precipitate pulmonary edema. It occasionally causes aseptic meningitis, and allograft thrombosis is reported three cases. It can also increase the incidence of post-transplant lymphoproliferative disorder (PTLD), especially when a positive donor is given to a negative recipient.

The common dosage is a 5- to 10-mg/dose, with premedication with steroids, acetaminophen, and benadryl. Each dose must be given slowly and the patient watched for signs of pulmonary edema. Duration of treatment is 10 to 14 days, for a total of 70 mg.

Interleukin-2 Receptor (CD25) Specific Monoclonal Antibodies

The receptor of IL-2 has three chains—alpha, beta, and gamma. The beta chain is induced with activation. The beta chain (or CD25) presence suggests prior T-cell activation. CD25 has been targeted to suppress activated cells and spare resting cells.

There are two commercially available CD25 molecules. Daclizumab (humanized anti-CD25 IgG1, Zenapax) and basiliximab (chimeric mouse–human anti-CD25 IgG1, Simulect). Both avoid immune clearance and can be used for prolonged periods without neutralizing antibody formation. These preparations avoid the serum sickness associated with mouse-, rabbit-, or horse-derived antibodies.

Alemtuzumab (Humanized Anti-CD52), Campath-1H

This is a humanized IgG1 derivative of rat antihuman CD52. CD52 is a nonmodulating glycosylphosphatidylinositol-anchored membrane protein with unknown function but high density on most T cells, B cells, and monocytes. Its main use is as an off-label induction agent. It works by rapidly depleting CD52-expressing lymphocytes centrally and peripherally in renal transplantation.

It allows for a delay in initiation of calcineurin inhibitor levels, which is good in DGF. It has been shown to be associated with an increase in antibody-mediated rejection or donor-specific antibody formation. Further studies are needed to determine its efficacy in rescue therapy.

Campath is administered as a 30-mg one-time dose. This one dose almost totally eliminates CD3 T cells within 1 hour, although secondary lymphoid depletion requires at least 48 hours and two doses. As with other antibodies, the patient should be premedicated prior to Campath for the cytokine release. There have been no neutralizing antibodies found to Campath.

Rituximab (Humanized Anti-CD20)

CD20 is a surface glycoprotein involved in B-cell activation and maturation, whose natural ligand is unknown. Rituximab was developed and approved for lymphogenous cancer and CD20+ B-cell lymphoma and PTLD. It has been suggested as a possible treatment for antibody-mediated rejection and rejection with vasculitis. It has also found a use in the sensitized patient to decrease antibodies to facilitate transplantation. The mechanism of action is thought to be depletional, primarily through inducing apoptosis.

Induction with rituximab is limited to donor specific sensitization with plasmapheresis, IVIG, or both. Rescue therapy with rituximab is investigational at this time. Its most important indication is primarily to treat PTLD.

Selected References

Braun F, et al. Update of current immunosuppressive drugs used in clinical organ transplantation. *Transpl Int.* 1998;*11*:77–81.

Gummert JF, et al. Newer immunosuppressive drugs: A review. *J Am Soc Nephrol.* 1999;*10*:1366–1380.

Haloran PF. Immunosuppressive drugs for kidney transplantation. *N Engl J Med.* 2004;*351*(26):2715–2729.

Morris PJ, Knechtle SJ. *Kidney transplantation principles and practice.* 6th ed. 2008: 220–332.

Sussman NL, Vierling JM. Overview of immunosuppression in adult liver transplantation. *UpToDate.* 2010.

Chapter 9

Infectious Complications After Abdominal Solid Organ Transplant

Federico Palacio and M. Hong Nguyen

Introduction

Solid organ transplantation is complicated by infections that pose serious threats to transplant recipients. The risk of infections, spectrum of infectious syndromes, and types of pathogens vary substantially according to the types of organ transplanted, surgical techniques used, immunosuppression regimen rendered, as well as the timeline of infections after transplant. In general, the risk of infection is determined by the immunosuppression status of the recipients, the epidemiological factors, and the administration of antimicrobial prophylaxis. In recent years there have been a number of changes in overall transplant practices that have altered the epidemiology of infectious complications. The broader use of antimicrobial prophylaxis for fungal, viral, and bacterial infections decreased the incidence of previously common infections, but new emergent resistant organisms have become more common.

This chapter discusses the immune status of abdominal organ transplant patients, the epidemiological exposures that predispose to infections after transplant, the timing of infection, and organ transplant-specific infection (kidney, liver, pancreas/kidney-pancreas, small intestine, and multivisceral transplant).

Immune Status of Abdominal Organ Transplant Recipients

Net state of immunosuppression is the term used to describe all possible risk factors that could be involved in the development of infection in a solid organ transplant (SOT) recipient. Factors that determine the net state of immunosuppression include immunosuppressive regimens, type of organ transplant and its associated technical complications, antimicrobial prophylaxis, viral co-infection (e.g., cytomegalovirus [CMV], Epstein-Barr virus [EBV], hepatitis C virus [HCV]), loss of the mucocutaneous barrier integrity, drug-induced leukopenia, and underlying diseases and comorbidities. The use of induction therapy at the time of transplant and the subsequent immunosuppressive regimens are by far the most important factors in determining the recipient's immune status. Table 9.1 summarizes the list of the most common classes of immunosuppressive agents and their potential effects on infections.

Table 9.1 Immunosuppressive Agents and Their Associated Risk of Infection

Classes of drugs	Drugs	Common side effects/toxicity	Common pathogens and their associated diseases
Calcineurin inhibitors	Cyclosporin	Nephrotoxicity, HTN, HLP, hirsutism, gingival hyperplasia	Polyoma-associated PML and PVAN PTLD Intracellular pathogens
	Tacrolimus	Neurotoxicity, glucose intolerance, alopecia, skin cancer	Gingival infection
Steroids	Prednisone, chronic	Poor wound healing	Pneumocystis, bacteria, molds, activation of hepatitis B and hepatitis C viruses
	Prednisone, bolus	Variable	CMV, polyomavirus nephropathy (PVAN)
Antimetabolite	Azathioprine	Leukopenia, thrombocytopenia, hepatotoxicity, gastrointestinal side effects	Papillomavirus
	Mycophenolate mofetil Mycophenolic acid sodium	Leukopenia, diarrhea	Early bacterial infection Delayed infection due to CMV infections, EBV and polyomavirus
Polyclonal antibody	ATGAM Thymoglobulin	Leukopenia, hypotension, myalgias, abdominal pain	Viruses (HSV, VZV, CMV, EBV-associated PTLD, BK PVAN). Fungi (especially when used to treat rejection rather than induction), including Pneumocystis. Accelerated HCV infection.
Monoclonal antibody	Muromonab-CD3 (OKT3)	Leukopenia, hypotension, myalgia, abdominal pain	Viruses (HSV, VZV, CMV, EBV, BK PVAN) Late fungal Increased hepatitis C replication
	Daclizumab Basiliximab	Edema, hypotension, anaphylaxis	Limited data, no evident effect

Classes of drugs	Drugs	Common side effects/toxicity	Common pathogens and their associated diseases
Cell cycle inhibitor	Sirolimus Everolimus	HLP, DVT, lymphocele, pancytopenia, TTP, HAT, hepatotoxicity, impaired wound healing	Pneumonitis (excess infections in combinations with calcineurin inhibitors)
Monoclonal antilymphocyte	Alemtuzumab (Belatacept, Bortezomib, Efalizumab, Eculizumab)	Prolonged lymphopenia	Viruses (HSV, VZV, CMV, BK PVAN, EBV-associated PTLD) Herpes virus Fungal infections (especially when used to treat rejection), including Pneumocystis. Potential for increased complications due to HBV and HCV.

HTN: hypertension; HLP: hyperlipidemia; PML: progressive multifocal leukoencephalopathy; PVAN: polyomavirus associated nephropathy PTLD: post-transplant lymphoproliferative disorder; CMV: cytomegalovirus; EBV: Epstein-Barr virus; ATGAM: lymphocyte immune globulin; DVT: deep venous thrombosis; TTP: thrombotic thrombocytopenic purpura; HAT: hepatic artery thrombosis.

Epidemiological Exposure

Epidemiological exposure includes four categories: donor-derived infections, recipient-derived infections, community-acquired infections, and nosocomial infections.

Donor-Derived Infections

In general, all potential organ donors undergo serological testing against Human immunodeficiency virus (HIV)-1 and -2, hepatitis B virus (HBV), HCV, CMV, EBV, Herpes simplex (HSV) and Varicella zoster viruses (VZV), syphilis, and *Toxoplasma gondii*. In addition, nucleic acid testing has been recently used to screen organs from high-risk lifestyle donors for HIV, HBV, and HCV. The Organ Procurement and Transplantation Network (OPTN) recommends to order other serology tests based on local epidemiology such as West Nile Virus (WNV) in areas with high local activity or *Trypanosoma cruzi* in California. As the result of this screening, donor-derived infections are rare events. However, when they occur, they are associated with high morbidity and mortality. To date, infections caused by viruses, bacteria, fungi, and parasites have all been linked to donor-derived infections (Table 9.2). Health-care workers should recognize that the classical signs and symptoms of infections of transplant recipients might be atypical because of their immunosuppressed status. Suspicion for donor-related infections should be heightened when clinical symptoms occur within 4–6 weeks after transplant and cannot be explained by the commonly encountered post-transplant complications, including nosocomial infections. When donor-derived infection is suspected, health-care workers should communicate rapidly to physicians from other transplant centers that received organs from the same donor, organ procurement organizations (OPOs), and public health authorities, as timely intervention (if it exists) might be life saving.

Table 9.2 Reported Donor-Derived Infections and Recommendations for Donor Screening

Etiological agents	Common clinical syndromes in transplant recipients	Donor screening recommended
Viruses		
HTLV-1 and -2	Subacute myelopathy, adult T-cell lymphoma/ leukemia, tropical spastic paraparesis.	Systemic screening in areas of high endemicity only*
West Nile virus (WNV)	Fever, neurological symptoms, encephalitis	-If donor is from areas of endemicity with active epidemic outbreak, or has aseptic meningitis or meningo-encephalitis, screen with NAT -Defer organ from donor with meningoencephalitic or myelitic symptoms of unknown etiology who resides in areas during periods of human WNV activity.
Rabies virus	Progressive neurological disease leading to coma and death; encephalitis	-If donor has a history of animal bite or exposure to bats, has unexplained mental or neurological symptoms, aseptic meninigitis or meningo-encephalitis, screen with serology (complement fixation test, enzyme linked immunosaasay); PCR; skin biopsy, saliva test, brain biopsy -Defer organs if the donor is at risk for rabies infection, and above tests cannot be performed
Lymphocytic choriomeningitis	Aseptic meningitis, encephalitis; unexplained fever, hepatitis, or multisystem organ failure.	If donor has aseptic meninigitis or meningoencephalitis, screen with PCR
Fungi		
Coccidioides immitis	Rapidly fatal, disseminated coccidioidomycosis.	If donor is from areas of endemicity, screen with serology (complement fixation and immunodiffusion).
Histoplasma capsulatum	Disseminated histoplasmosis.	If donor is from areas of endemicity, or radiologic findings suggestive of active or past histoplasmosis, screen with serology.
Cryptococcus neoformans	Cryptococcal fungemia, pneumonia, encephalitis.	No firm recommendations, but consider infections due to C. neoformans in patients with unexplained neurologic symptoms.

Etiological agents	Common clinical syndromes in transplant recipients	Donor screening recommended
Parasites		
Toxoplasma gondii (rare in abdominal transplant)	Ocular infection, central nervous system, disseminated toxoplasmosis.	Evaluate donor and recipient Toxoplasma serology; consider prophylaxis for patients with D+/R- and R+.
Plasmodium spp.	Thrombocytopenia, neurological symptoms, coma.	If donor had traveled to areas of endemicity within 3 preceding years, screen with thick and thin blood smears or PCR before accepting organs.
Trypanosoma cruzi	Asymptomatic parasitemia, acute infection with fever and hepatosplenomegaly, chagasic myocarditis	If donor is from areas of endemicity, screen with serology or PCR.
Strongyloides stercoralis	Rash, gastro-intestinal symptoms, hyperinfection syndrome.	If donor had traveled to areas of endemicity within 3 preceding years, screen with serology
Others		
Mycobacterium tuberculosis	Pulmonary, extrapulmonary, disseminated tuberculosis.	-Defer organ from donors with active TB -Living donor should have tuberculin skin test or Quantiferon TB Gold performed; donor with +test should be treated for latent TB prior to organ donation -Recipient of organ from donor with known +tuberculin skin test or Quantiferon TB Gold test should receive INH prophylaxis

* Enzyme immune-assay for HILV-1/-2 is currently not available. Based on the extremely low incidence of HTLV-1/-2 among blood donors in the United States (<0.05%), the OPTN/UNOS Board of Directors voted to discontinue the requirement to perform prospective screening of deceased donors in 2009.

NAT: nucleic acid tests; PCR: polymerase chain reaction INH: Isoniazid.

Recipient-Derived Infections

In general, a detailed medical history, and, infectious diseases, vaccination, remote and recent travel, and behavioral history should be obtained before transplantation to identify potential risk factors for infections post-transplantation. In addition, serology screening for recipients should be performed just in the case of high-risk donors. The screening results from donors and recipients are paired (especially against CMV, EBV, and *T. gondii*) to determine risk stratification for antimicrobial prophylaxis after transplant. Infections after transplantation are typically related to colonization or infection just before transplantation. Active infections need to be eliminated in transplant recipients, if possible, before transplantation, because immunosuppression can aggravate previous or active infections.

Community-Acquired Infections

Transplant recipients once in the community are at risk for community-acquired infections, similarly to the general population. Infections in the organ transplant patients, when compared to the general population, however, are more frequent and associated with more severe disease and higher mortality rates. For example, the risk for invasive pneumococcal infections is 12.8-fold higher in transplant recipients compared to the general population. In addition, the morbidity and mortality of organ transplant patients resulting from influenza A H1N1 in 2009 was more substantial than in the general population, with 71% requiring hospitalization, 16% requiring admission to intensive care units (ICUs), and a mortality rate of 4%. These community-acquired infections, although occurring later after transplant, also predispose patients to rejection. Common community-acquired bacterial pathogens include *Streptococcus pneumoniae*, *Legionella spp*, *Mycoplasma pneumoniae*, *Listeria monocytogenes*, and *Salmonella spp*. Common viral pathogens include influenza, parainfluenza, respiratory syncitial virus (RSV), adenovirus, and human metapneumovirus. Endemic fungi such as *Coccidioides immitis*, *Histoplasma capsulatum*, *Blastomyces dermatitidis*, or environmental fungi such as *Cryptococcous neoformans* and *Aspergillus spp*. may also cause infection while the patients are in the community.

Nosocomial Infections

Transplant recipients are at high risk for nosocomial infections from prolonged mechanical ventilation and/or hospitalization after transplantation, surgical complications, and their immunosuppressed status. They are also at risk for colonization and infection with multiple-drug-resistant (MDR) organisms. Recent reports have documented an increase in antimicrobial-resistant organisms that afflict organ transplant recipients, among which are vancomycin-resistant *Enterococcus* (VRE), MDR or pan-drug resistant Gram–negative rods, and *Clostridium difficile*. The epidemiology of these resistant organisms is summarized below.

Clostridium Difficile Infection

The incidence of *C. difficile* infection (CDI) among organ transplant patients is higher than the nontransplant population (1%–2%) and varies according to the organs transplanted: kidney and heart transplantation is associated with the lowest rates (1%–16%), whereas intestinal (9%), liver (3%–7%), and lung (7%–31%) have the highest rates. CDI is most prominent during the first 3 months after transplant, although late infections are also a problem. Up to thirteen percent of organ transplant patients with CDI develop fulminant colitis, but the overall mortality of CDI is not higher than nontransplant patients. The typical risk factors for CDI in the general population are also applied to organ transplant patients. In addition, immunosuppression, hypo-gamma-globulinemia that is commonly associated with lung, heart and liver transplants, and the routine use of agents for gastric acid suppression such as proton pump inhibitor and H_2 receptor antagonist also predispose organ transplant patients to CDI. The best means to prevent CDI in organ transplant patients are limiting broad spectrum antibiotic use, avoidance of H_2 blocker or proton pump inhibitors, and strict hand hygiene to prevent nosocomial spread. There is no known effective antimicrobial prophylaxis against CDI, and the use of probiotics is not recommended because of lack of efficacy and safety data for organ transplant patients.

Infections Caused by Enterococcus spp.

Enterococcus is a commonly encountered pathogen after abdominal transplant, causing bloodstream, intra-abdominal, urinary tract, and wound infections. Paralleling the general trend worldwide, VRE has emerged among organ transplant patients. The prevalence of VRE colonization and infection among liver and kidney recipients is between 3% to 55% and 4% to 11%, respectively. Longitudinal studies in liver transplant patients showed that 32% of patients colonized before transplant went on to develop VRE infection after transplant. In addition, 18% of liver transplant patients acquired VRE colonization after transplant, and these patients fared much worse than those colonized with VRE before transplantation. Overall, VRE infections in transplant patients are associated with persistent and recurrent infections, utilization of more hospital resources, and higher mortality rates.

Infections Caused by Multidrug Resistant (MDR) Gram negative rods

Over the past decade, there have been increasing trends of colonization and infections with MDR Gram–negative bacteria in organ transplant patients. These include extended spectrum β-lactamases (ESBL) producing enteric organisms, *Klebsiella pneumoniae* carbapenemase (KPC)-producing Enterobacteria, and extended- or pan-drug resistant *Acinetobacter baumannii*. For example, surveillance data in 1998 showed that 22% and 54% of liver and intestinal transplant recipients, respectively, were colonized with ESBL-producing *Klebsiella spp.* Reports of infections caused by AmpC β-lactamase and ESBL-producing Gram–negative rods as well as KPC also emerged, especially in the kidney, kidney-pancreas, and liver transplant recipients. In addition, sporadic nosocomial outbreaks resulting from these resistant organisms have also been recognized. Extended- and pan-drug resistant *Acinetobacter baumannii* is also an important pathogen in the organ transplant recipients, but this pathogen mostly affects lung and heart-lung transplant patients. Infections caused by resistant Gram–negative rods carry a high morbidity and mortality, given lack of effective therapy. In addition, failure of therapy and/or emergence of resistance during therapy with tigecycline and colistin (the two most commonly used agents for treatment of extensive drug and pan drug resistant Gram negative rods infection) have been reported.

Timing of Infection Post-Transplantation

After solid organ transplantation, the timeline of infection is divided in three periods when specific infections typically occur: early post-transplantation period (0–1 month), intermediate post-transplantation period (1–6 months), and late post-transplantation period (>6 months). In general, during the early period, the most common infections are surgical- or nosocomial-related. During the intermediate period, infections result from re-activation of latent organisms or opportunistic pathogens. Finally, during the late period, community-acquired pathogens including bacteria, viruses, and fungi predominate. The use of this timeline assists physicians in developing differential diagnosis while evaluating patients post-transplant, as well as in selecting antimicrobial prophylaxis regimens. It should be pointed out that infections outside these timelines are still possible, especially in patients with chronic rejection that requires more prolonged or more potent immunosuppressive regimens. As long as the immunosuppression is still significant, the patients remain prone to opportunistic infections, regardless of the timeline, post-transplantation. Therefore, the timeline should be reset every time an immunosuppression regimen is intensified. Table 9.3 summarizes the common opportunistic pathogens, their timeline of infection, clinical syndromes, and recommended prophylaxis and interventions.

Early Post-Transplantation Period (0–1 Month)

During the first month post-transplantation, infections are similar to those observed in any surgical patients, although they might be more frequent and more severe given the immunosuppression. At this stage, the net state of immunosuppression has not been prolonged enough to favor opportunistic infections. The transplanted organs and surgical techniques largely determine the spectrum of infection (please refer to Organ Transplant-Specific Infections section below). In this early period, surgical-related infections are the most important, but other nosocomial infections such as hospital-acquired or ventilator-associated pneumonia, catheter-related bloodstream infections, antibiotic-associated diarrhea, and catheter-related urinary tract infections might also occur. Finally, donor-derived infections and recipient-derived infections discussed above also contribute to these early onset infections.

Bacteria

The predominant organisms causing infections during this period are nosocomial bacteria that are encountered at individual local hospitals, such as *Staphylococcus aureus*, a variety of Gram–negative rods, *C. difficile*, and *Legionella spp.*, as well as endogenous bacteria originating from surgical wound or anastomotic sites, such as *Enterococcus spp.*, Gram–negative enteric organisms, and *Candida spp.*

Fungi

Fungal infections during the first month post-abdominal transplantation are mainly due to *Candida spp.*, which is strongly influenced by surgical factors. Besides the classical risk factors for invasive candidiasis such as broad spectrum antibiotics, central venous catheters, and acute renal failure requiring dialysis, the following factors predispose to invasive candidiasis in organ transplant recipients: primary graft failure, surgical re-exploration, and Candida colonization. In addition, specific surgical techniques also predispose to invasive candidiasis e.g.,

Table 9.3 Timeline of Infection After Organ Transplantation

	Early onset (<1 month)	Intermediate onset (1–6 months)	Late onset (>6 months)
Organisms			
Bacteria	Nosocomial bacteria, including MRSA, VRE, MDR Gram-negative, *C. difficile*	*Nocardia spp, Listeria spp* Nosocomial bacteria *Mycobacterium tuberculosis*	Community-acquired bacteria *Nocardia*
Fungi	*Candida spp* (predominant) *Aspergillus spp* (uncommon)	-PCP (if not receiving prophylaxis) -*Aspergillus* -Endemic fungi	Molds *Cryptococcus neoformans* Endemic fungi
Viruses	Recipient-derived: HSV, HBV, HCV	-CMV, HSV, VZV (if not receiving prophylaxis) -EBV, HHV-6, HHV-7 -BK polymyomavirus -HBV, HCV -Adenovirus, influenza	-Delayed CMV (especially in patients with mismatch D+/R-) -HSV, VZV -EBV-associated PTLD -HBV, HCV -Community-acquired respiratory viruses -JC Polymyomavirus
Parasites	*T. cruzi*	*Strongyloides stercoralis, T. gondii, Leishmania, T. cruzi*	
Types of infections			
Types of infection	Nosocomial Wound infection Pneumonia Catheter-associated Bacteremia UTI *C. difficile* infection	Opportunistic infection Nosocomial infections: - (as in early onset) - Respiratory viruses	Opportunistic infection Community-acquired: - Pneumonia - UTI	Community-acquired pneumonia or UTI Opportunistic infections (if recipient is being maintained on high level of immunosuppression)

(continued)

Table 9.3 (Continued)

	Early onset (<1 month)	Intermediate onset (1–6 months)	Late onset (>6 months)
Donor-derived infections	- graft-associated viral infections (LCMV, WNV, rabies, HIV) - graft-associated parasitic infections (T. cruzi)	*Mycobacterium tuberculosis* Endemic fungus *Strongyloides stercoralis*, *T. gondii*, *Leishmania*, *T. cruzi*	-CMV, EBV, HBV, HCV
Recipient-derived infections	-bacteria (MRSA, VRE, Gram–negative bacteria) -fungi (*Candida spp, Aspergillus spp*)	*Mycobacterium tuberculosis* Endemic fungus	-CMV, HSV, VZV, HBV, HCV
Sources of organisms	-Nosocomial -Recipient (endogenous, colonization, reactivation) Donor	Recipient (reactivation, colonization) Donor transmission Nosocomial Community	
Predisposing factors			
Risk factors	Nosocomial infections Surgical-related Anastomotic complications Reperfusion injury	Intense immunosuppressive therapy Nosocomial infections (if patients remain hospitalized) Surgical-related Anastomotic complications	Immunosuppressive therapy Community infections

choledochojejunostomy in liver transplant and enteric drainage in pancreatic transplant. Prophylaxis with anti-candida antifungal agent should be considered for patients with these risk factors.

Historically, invasive aspergillosis has occurred in the early period after transplant, but recent studies have shown that the timeline has shifted to the intermediate period. Advances in surgical techniques, the use of effective prophylaxis against CMV leading to delayed-onset CMV infection, and graft dysfunction or failure caused by recurrent HCV infection are thought to be factors influencing this shift in timeline. For liver transplant recipients, risk factors for invasive aspergillosis include re-transplantation and renal failure requiring dialysis, which confer a 30-fold and 15- to 25-fold higher risk, respectively. Other risk factors such as fulminant hepatic failure as the indication for transplant, and intra-abdominal or thoracic re-exploration within the first month after transplantation also predispose patients to invasive aspergillosis. Invasive aspergillosis carries a high rate of morbidity and mortality—especially shortly after liver transplant—and prophylaxis with a mold-effective antifungal agent should be considered for patients harboring these risk factors.

Infections resulting from fungi other than Candida, such as *Cryptococcus neoformans*, and endemic fungi caused by *Blastomyces dermatitidis*, *Histoplasma capsulatum*, and *Coccidioides immitis* are rare during this period but have been reported.

Viruses
Viral pathogens rarely cause problems in this period. If they occur, the pathogens are either HSV or viruses derived from donor graft (e.g., Lymphocytic Choriomeningitis Virus (LCMV), WNV, rabies, HIV). The incidence of HSV infection has markedly diminished since the widespread use of anti-viral prophylaxis after transplant.

Parasites
Parasitic pathogens rarely cause disease during this stage, but donor-derived infections resulting from *T. cruzi*, *Strongyloides stercoralis*, *Plasmodium spp.*, *Balamuthia mandrillaris*, or *Toxoplasma* have been reported (Table 9.2).

Intermediate Post-Transplantation Period (1–6 Months)
During this period, transplant recipients reach the highest net state of immunosuppression, thus are prone to developing opportunistic infections. However, remaining complications from the peri-operative period and donor- and recipient-derived infections can still persist. Nosocomial infections are also a problem if the recipients remain hospitalized. In general, the geographical and epidemiological factors, immunosuppression regimen, and antimicrobial prophylaxis at individual institutions all influence the rates and types of opportunistic infections observed during this period.

Viral Pathogens
Without antiviral prophylaxis, the most common causes of fever during this period are either due to viral infections or allograft rejection. Members of the Herpes viruses are now less common with the use of prophylaxis but remain a

major problem at centers where universal antiviral prophylaxis is not applied. Other viruses, including BK Polyomavirus (please refer to Specific Infections After Kidney Transplant section below), HBV, and HCV, can reactivate.

Cytomegalovirus infection occurs in approximately 19% of organ transplant recipients. The most important risk factor for CMV infection is the receipt of organ from a donor with CMV-seropositive into a recipient with CMV-seronegative before transplant (CMV D+/R-). The other risk factors include graft rejection requiring immunosuppression augmentation, concomitant viral infections resulting from Human herpes virus-6 and -7 (HHV-6 and HHV-7), and the use of antibody against lymphocyte. Lung, intestine, and kidney-pancreas transplants are associated with a higher risk for CMV infection than liver, heart, and kidney transplant. Among organ transplants, the rates of CMV infection among R+ and D+/R- are 6% and 45%, respectively, for renal transplant; 18% and 44%, respectively, for liver transplant; and 62% and 62%, respectively, for intestinal transplant.

Despite advances in antiviral prophylaxis and treatment, infections caused by CMV remain a major problem in organ transplant population. Cytomegalovirus exerts both direct effects on organs to cause diseases as well as indirect effects that threaten allograft function, predispose patients to infection, and worsen mortality. Cytomegalovirus infection encompasses a wide spectrum of clinical manifestations ranging from asymptomatic CMV viremia and CMV syndrome (febrile illness in the setting of CMV viremia) to organ-invasive CMV disease. In organ transplant patients, the most common organ involved is the transplanted allograft organ—that is, pneumonia in lung transplant patients, hepatitis in liver transplant patients, pancreatitis in pancreas transplant patients, colitis in intestine transplant patients, and nephritis in renal transplant patients. The indirect effect of CMV is exerted by modulating the immune system, leading to increasing risk of infections caused by bacteria, virus (EBV, HHV-6, HHV-7, and HCV), and fungi as well as lymphoproliferative disease. Active CMV replication has been associated with both acute and chronic allograft rejection, such as accelerated vasculopathy in heart transplant and bronchiolitis obliterans syndrome in lung transplant, and allograft dysfunction, such as vanishing bile duct syndrome in liver transplant, and tubulo-interstitial fibrosis and glomerulopathy after kidney transplant.

Given the negative impact of CMV, efforts have been made to prevent CMV in organ transplantation. There are two general approaches: universal prophylaxis and preemptive therapy. The advantages and disadvantages of these approaches are summarized in Table 9.4. The duration of preemptive therapy is approximately 3 months, whereas the duration of universal prophylaxis is unclear. In general, prophylaxis is recommended for 3 months for kidney, liver, and pancreas and 6 months for intestinal transplant for CMV-seropositive recipients pre-transplant. The duration of prophylaxis for D+/R- is at least 6 months. To date, the approaches to prophylaxis are transplanted organ- and institutional-dependent. Data to date favor the use of universal prophylaxis over preemptive therapy in the highest risk transplant patients (CMV D+/R-). The major limitation to this approach, besides drug cost and toxicity, is the development of delayed-onset CMV infection, especially among the patients with CMV D+/R-. It has become clear that in a subset of patients, antiviral prophylaxis does not

Table 9.4 Advantages and Disadvantages of Universal Prophylaxis Versus Preemptive Therapy for CMV Infection After Organ Transplant (adapted from Humar A, Snydman D. Cytomegalovirus in solid organ transplant recipients. *Am J Transplant* 2009 Dec;9 Suppl 4:S78-86.

	Universal prophylaxis	Preemptive therapy
Definition	Administer antiviral to all patients at risk for CMV	Administer antiviral therapy only if there is evidence of CMV replication
Ease of approach	Easy to coordinate	Time and effort of staff CMV test is not standardized
Cost	Drug cost	Lab monitoring cost
Efficacy	Prevents CMV disease	Prevents CMV disease
Toxicity	Potential higher bone marrow toxicity	Potential lower drug toxicity
Late-onset disease	Potential problem	Less than with prophylaxis
Indirect effects	Less rates of graft loss Less opportunistic infection Higher graft survival	

eliminate but only delays CMV infection. In general, delayed-onset CMV occurs in 29% to 37% of patients within 3 months of drug discontinuation. The risk factors for delayed-onset CMV are CMV D+/R-, allograft rejection, and higher immunosuppression. Late-onset CMV infection is independently associated with increased overall mortality at 1 year.

Epstein-Barr virus (EBV) affects closed to 90% of adult patients. It is transmitted via oral secretions, and establishes latency in resting memory B cells. Epstein-Barr virus-specific cytotoxic T cells are depressed in the setting of chronic immunosuppression, which in turn promotes uncontrolled EBV-driven B-cell proliferation and tumor formation. Epstein-Barr virus-associated post-transplant lymphoproliferative disease (PTLD) occurs in approximately 15% of organ transplant recipients. Eighty percent of PTLD occurring within 1 year after transplant is of B-cell origin. The most important risk factor for EBV-associated PTLD is EBV mismatch status of EBV-seronegative recipient receiving an organ from an EBV-seropositive donor. Other risk factors include organ transplanted and types and intensity of immunosuppression. The incidence of PTLD is highest among intestinal transplant (31%), lung (3.8% to 11.7%), and liver (6.8%–13.1%) transplant patients and less in kidney transplant patients (1.2%–9%). Cytomegalovirus infection and chronic HCV infection might also predispose organ transplant patients to PTLD. There is a wide clinical presentation of EBV, ranging from benign Polyclonal B-Cell Monononucleosis syndrome with fever and weight loss to malignant, monoclonal lymphoma. Most patients develop extranodal solid tumors, but PTLD can also involve the allograft. The mortality rate for adult patients with PTLD is close to 50%. There is currently no universally acceptable preventive strategy. Because high EBV viral load often antedates PTLD, several institutions apply preemptive therapy for high-risk patients, but to date, there are insufficient data to suggest the best approach. Therapy for PTLD remains a challenge, and reduction of immunosuppression is key because this may result in the regression of PTLD in up to 50% of patients. Adjunctive therapy includes surgical resection of the tumor with or without local irradiation, monoclonal B-cell antibody therapy with rituximab, and cytotoxic chemotherapy.

Fungal Pathogens

During this period of intense and peaked immunosuppression, organ transplant recipients are at high risk for fungal mold infections, especially *A. fumigatus*. Invasive aspergillosis occurs in 1% to 15%, and the incidence depends on the type of organ transplanted. The incidence is highest for intestinal transplant patients (0%–10%) and liver transplant patients (1%–8%) and lowest for kidney (0%–4%). In a prospective study by the Transplant-Associated Infection Surveillance Network (TRANSNET), the cumulative incidence of invasive aspergillosis was 0.7%, whereas the cumulative incidence of cryptococcosis, mold infections other than aspergillosis and zygomycosis, and endemic fungal infections was only 0.2%. A noteworthy finding from this study is that there was a difference in the incidence of fungal infections among participating sites, which was speculated to result from variability in complexity and acuity of transplant recipients, surgical technique, antifungal prophylaxis and empirical treatment strategies, immunosuppressive regimens, and approach to diagnosis.

Pneumocystis pneumonia (PCP) resulting from *Pneumocystis jiroveci* occurred in 5% to 15% of organ transplant recipients before the era of universal prophylaxis. Trimethoprim-sulfamethoxazole is very effective in preventing infections and is recommended for at least 6 to 12 months after transplantation.

Endemic mycosis including *Histoplasma capsulatum*, *Coccidioides immitis*, and less frequently *Blastomyces dermatitidis* may reactivate during this period, but the infections mostly appear 6 months after transplant.

Table 9.5 summarizes the clinical characteristics of common opportunistic infections after organ transplantation, and the current recommendations for prophylaxis.

Parasitic Pathogens

Toxoplasmosis during this period is usually prevented by the use of trimethoprim-sulfamethoxazole prophylaxis. Reactivation of latent parasitic infections like Chagas disease and Strongyloidiasis have been observed. Gastrointestinal parasites like Cryptosporidium and Microsporidium may cause diarrhea during this period.

Late Post-Transplant Period (>6 Months)

Beyond 6 months, most patients are out in the community and receive basal level of immunosuppression, so they are at low risk for opportunistic infections. However, similarly to the general population, these patients are subjected to

Table 9.5 Description of Common Opportunistic Infections and Recommended Prophylaxis

	Rates of infection without prophylaxis* and onset of infection after transplant	Risk factors	Common clinical manifestations	Recommend prophylaxis
Viruses				
CMV	D-/R-: <5% R+: 6%–18% D+/R-: 44% 1–6 months (delayed CMV infection occurs in patients receiving antiviral prophylaxis)	Immunosuppression, acute rejection, advanced age, and poor kidney transplant graft function. Small intestine and pancreas transplant have the highest risks for CMV infection among the abdominal transplant	-Asymptomatic CMV viremia -CMV syndrome -CMV disease	Universal prophylaxis or preemptive treatment Also prevents HSV and VZV infections
HSV	40%–50% to 75% Reactivation occurs in the first 6 months (mostly within 3 weeks) Primary infection occurs any time	Lymphocyte antibody induction, mycophenolate	-oral or genital mucocutaneous lesions -organ disease: hepatitis, pneumonia, disseminated visceral disease	Prophylaxis for >1 month after transplant Additional prophylaxis against HSV is not needed during active CMV prophylaxis
VZV	1%–12% Reactivation occurs 4–23 months after transplant Primary infection occurs any time	Risk factors not well defined. Older transplant recipients, more intense immunosuppression, mycophenolate mofetil	-dermatomal vesicular rash -visceral dissemination	Prophylaxis for >1 month Additional prophylaxis against HSV is not needed during active CMV prophylaxis

(continued)

Table 9.5 (Continued)

	Rates of infection without prophylaxis* and onset of infection after transplant	Risk factors	Common clinical manifestations	Recommend prophylaxis
EBV	Primary EBV: 6 weeks Reactivation EBV: 2–3 months Highest in the first year after transplant	-early PTLD (<12 months): primary EBV infection, young age, types of organ transplant, CMV mismatch or disease, antibody induction -late PTLD (>12 months) duration of immunosuppression, type of organ transplant, older age	-infectious mononucleosis -hepatitis, pneumonitis, GI symptoms and hematological diseases -PTLD	Role of prophylaxis is unclear Preemptive therapy and lower immunosuppression
Mycobacterium tuberculosis				
Mycobacterium tuberculosis	1%–6% (developed countries), 15% in endemic areas Median: 9 months (reactivation occurs within 1 year in two-thirds of patients)	Positive tuberculin skin test, travel to areas endemic for TB, receipt of T-cell-depleting antibodies, old age	-pulmonary TB -extrapulmonary TB -disseminated TB	Treatment for latent TB is recommended for: 1. + tuberculin skin test or + Quantiferon TB Gold; 2. radiographic evidence of previous TB; 3. received donor with tuberculin test +; 4. history of close contact with individual with active TB.

Dimorphic fungi			
Histoplasma capsulatum	0.4%–2% Median: 17 mos 2 mos–7 yrs		Pulmonary Hepatomegaly and splenomegaly (25%–60%) CNS involvement (10%) Septic shock, skin, mucous membranes, adrenal, bone, pancreatitis, pericarditis, pyelonephritis, bone marrow involvement Disseminated (75%)	Serology screen before transplant not recommended because of low likelihood for infection Secondary prophylaxis might be considered for those with active histoplasmosis during the 2 years before transplant
Coccidioides immitis	3%–9% 50% <3 months 70% <1 year	Acute rejection History of coccidioidomycosis or (+) pre-transplant serology	Pulmonary Cutaneous, osteo-articular, CNS Disseminated (75%)	Travel history Primary antifungal prophylaxis for donor or recipient with history of coccidioidomycosis or serology +
Blastomyces dermatitidis	0.14% 12 days–250 months 55% >2 years	Not clearly defined because of small case series.	-pulmonary; 67% complicated by Acute Respiratory Distress Syndrome ARDS -extrapulmonary sites: skin, soft tissue, fungemia -Disseminated (48%)	Serology tests not yet perfected Primary or secondary prophylaxis not recommended

(continued)

Table 9.5 (Continued)

	Rates of infection without prophylaxis* and onset of infection after transplant	Risk factors	Common clinical manifestations	Recommend prophylaxis
Other fungi				
Aspergillus spp.	1%–15% <1 month–6 months	Retransplantation and renal failure requiring dialysis	Pulmonary, extrapulmonary, CNS, disseminated aspergillosis	Targeted prophylaxis may be considered for patients s/p retransplantation or re-operation, renal failure requiring dialysis, transplantation for fulminant hepatic failure.
Cryptococcus neoformans	0.3%–5% >6 months	antibody against lymphocyte for induction; treatment of rejection	CNS, pulmonary, fungemia, disseminated	Prophylaxis not indicated
Pneumocystis spp	2% to 10%–15% 1–6 months	Antibody induction, calcineurin inhibitors, prolonged use of steroid, CMV disease	Pneumonia (interstitial pneumonia is more common)	Universal prophylaxis for >6–12 months. Also prevent most infections caused by T. gondii, and Listeria. monocytogenes

* Rates of opportunistic infections vary with the types of organ transplant and the immunosuppression regimen.

Among abdominal transplant patients, lifelong prophylaxis for PCP is recommended for small bowel transplant, patients with a history of prior PCP infection or chronic CMV disease. Lifelong prophylaxis is also recommended for patients on intensified immunosuppression.

community-acquired infections resulting from bacteria, viruses, and fungi (see Community-Acquired Infections section above). Reactivation of latent viruses that were previously suppressed by antiviral prophylaxis (such as Herpes Zoster and CMV) can occur during this period when the prophylaxis is discontinued. Other viral infections like HBV, HCV, and EBV may also emerge.

Infections resulting from *Mycobacterium tuberculosis*, endemic mycosis, and aspergillosis peak during this late period. Depending on disease prevalence, the rates of tuberculosis after organ transplant range from 0.35% to 15%. Infections due to other less common fungi such as *Zygomycetes*, *Fusarium*, *Scedosporium*, and *dematiaceous molds (Exophiala spp, Alternaria spp, Dactylaria spp, Cladophialophora spp, Curvularia spp*, etc.) are also observed. Most patients with these fungal infections have unique risk factors such as neutropenia, poorly controlled diabetes mellitus, malnutrition, renal failure, and heightened immunosuppression. Although rare, donor-derived *H. capsulatum* infections diagnosed after 6 months of transplant have also been described. Cryptococcosis affects 0.3% to 5% of abdominal transplant patients, and typically occurs 6 months after transplant. Of note, cryptococcosis occurs relatively earlier among liver transplant recipients (<12 months) than among those who receive other organs (16–21 months). The use of antibodies against lymphocyte for induction and treatment of rejection are risk factors. Cryptococcosis disseminates to the central nervous system or to extrapulmonary sites in 53% to 72% of patients; liver transplant recipients have the highest risk for dissemination.

Patients suffers from chronic rejection requiring repeated courses of intensified immunosuppressive therapy or a higher basal level of immunosuppression are at higher risk for opportunistic infections jiroveci and more severe infections from community pathogens. More prolonged prophylaxis for PCP in these patients is indicated.

Organ Transplant-Specific Infections

In addition to infections commonly seen in all organ transplantation, each type of organ transplantation is associated with a set of technical and medical problems, which predispose to a unique set of infectious complications. These organ-specific infections are discussed below.

Specific Infections After Kidney Transplantation

Urinary tract infection (UTI) is the most common bacterial infection in kidney transplant recipients, occurring in up to 86% of patients. UTI mostly occurs within the first 3 months after transplant. Risk factors for UTI includes presence of indwelling bladder catheter, female gender, advanced age, diabetes mellitus, polycystic kidney disease, history of immunosuppression, vesicoureteral reflux, and history of recurrent UTIs, and prolonged period of dialysis before transplantation (especially peritoneal). Technical complications of transplant including ureteral anastomosis, placement of intra-operative ureteral stents, and allograft trauma also predispose to UTIs after transplant. The etiological agents are similar to those causing UTIs in the general population, but MDR organisms (including *Pseudomonas aeruginosa* and *Enterococcus spp*) and *Candida spp.* have emerged as significant pathogens. Urinary tract infections after transplant might manifest in many different ways, ranging from asymptomatic bacteriuria and uncomplicated cystitis to more severe infections like graft-site candidiasis, acute allograft pyelonephritis, or emphysematous pyelonephritis. Early onset UTIs are associated with a higher rate of complications (pyelonephritis, bacteremia, or relapse) than late-onset UTIs that develop more than 6 months after transplant. Indeed, late-onset UTIs are generally uncomplicated and, when associated with bacteremia or recurrent infection, should prompt investigation for anatomic or functional abnormalities. Urinary tract infections, either early or late onset after transplantation, are associated with poor graft outcomes.

Wound infection is the most common surgical-related complications after renal transplantation. Superficial wound infections are usually secondary to skin contamination, and deep wound infections are usually related with infected urinary leaks. Risk factors for wound complications include obesity, older age of donor or recipient, and diabetes mellitus. Other surgical complications that might predispose to infections are vascular (vein or artery thrombosis/stenosis), and urological complications (e.g., urinomas, obstruction, lymphoceles, hematuria). Urinomas rarely become infected, but when they occur, they are caused by members of the *Enterobacteriaceae* group of bacteria.

Graft-site candidiasis is a rare complication, with an incidence of 1 per 1000 renal transplants. It manifests as renal or iliac arteritis, isolated graft-site abscess, infected urinoma, or surgical site infections. If candidemia occurs early after transplant, then candida arteritis or renal aneurysm should be considered, as it is associated with poor outcomes and requires nephrectomy in 50% to 70% of the cases. It is important to point out that a negative blood culture for Candida does not rule out Candida graft-site infection or arteritis.

Bacteremia is also an important complication after renal transplant. Sixty percent of bacteremias originate from or around the urinary tract, and 50% of the bacteremic UTIs are associated with technical complications related to surgery such as ureteral leaks, stricture, or perinephric hematoma.

Polyomavirus resulting from BK and, to a lesser extent, JC, is an important cause of graft loss in renal transplant patients. Similarly to the herpes viruses, BK establishes latency after primary infection; the sites of latency are renal cortex, medulla, urothelial cells, and bladder. BK virus reactivates after renal transplant and affects 10% to 60% of patients. Most of the reactivation occurs during the first year post-transplantation, and the site of the reactivation determines the presentation: ureteral stenosis if reactivation occurs in the ureter and hemorrhagic cystitis if reactivation occurs in the bladder. If reactivation is within the kidney, BK virus-associated nephropathy (PVAN) ensues, which commonly manisfests as worsening in creatinine. The diagnosis of PVAN requires a renal biopsy demonstrating intranuclear viral inclusions with inflammation and is confirmed with immunohistochemistry or *in situ* hybridization. It is standard practice to monitor viral replication in the urine (decoy cells or polymerase chain reaction [PCR]) at least every 3 months during the first 2 years after transplant, then yearly until the fifth year. BK viruria should trigger testing for BK in plasma. A positive plasma viremia, especially when persistent, should prompt reduction in immunosuppressive therapy. Using this monitoring, 80% to 90% of patients at risk for PVAN can be identified before significant PVAN develops. Drug therapy against PVAN is limited. Cidofovir and leflunomide have activity against BK in vitro. Cidofovir shows promise when combined with lower immunosuppression but is limited by nephrotoxicity. The overall prognosis for graft survival after PVAN is poor; 1% to 4% of graft loss is related to BK virus disease.

Infections After Liver Transplantation

Over the last decade, despite the improvement in surgical techniques with reduction in operative time and progress in immunosuppressive medications, the rate of infectious complications remains high (ranging from 54% to 67%), and infection and sepsis remain the most common cause of death Indeed, liver transplantation is a complex surgical procedure with a high rate of post-surgical complications and infections. For example, Roux-en-Y choledochojejunostomy is associated with a higher risk of biliary complications (biliary stenosis, leaks, and infectious cholangitis). Hepatic artery thrombosis (HAT), affecting 2% to 11% of the recipients after liver transplantation, is associated with high rates of graft loss, infections such as cholangitis, recurrent hepatic abscesses and bacteremia, and increased mortality. Patients transplanted for primary biliary cirrhosis have a high rate of post-operative biliary complications that lead to anastomotic stricture and bacterial cholangitis post-transplantation.

The most consistently identified risk factors for infections in the post-operative period are:

- Duration of surgery
- Retransplantation
- Intra-operative blood transfusions
- Intraperitoneal blood
- Prolonged total ischemia time

Surgical-site infections affect approximately 32% of liver transplant recipients. Peritonitis, intrahepatic abscesses, and cholangitis are the most common infections, accounting for 27% to 48% of all bacterial infections early after transplant. Peritonitis and abscesses may complicate biliary leaks, which is especially common after living donor transplant. These infections are often polymicrobial with MDR enteric Gram–negative bacteria spp as well as anaerobes and *Candida spp.* Multidrug-resistant Gram–positive bacteria (VRE, MRSA) are also common in liver transplant recipients, especially when selective bowel decontamination is used.

Bilomas occurred in approximately 12% of patients after liver transplant. These are intrahepatic or perihepatic fluid collections that develop as complications of HAT or stenosis, biliary necrosis, stricture, or leaks. Nosocomial MDR

Gram–positive bacteria such as VRE and *Candida spp.* are the most pathogens, followed by MDR Gram–negative bacteria. Coagulase-negative *Staphylococcus* is also an important pathogen, especially when bilomas are associated with T-tube drainage. If bilomas are associated with HAT, then retransplantation is usually required.

Candida spp affects 53% to 68% of liver recipients and is the most common cause of invasive fungal infection. Candid a bloodstream infection and intra-abdominal abscess are the most common infections caused by *Candida spp.* followed by peritonitis, esophagitis, and disseminated disease. Risk factors for invasive candidiasis includes choledochojejunostomy, prolonged operative time (≥11 hours) requiring substantial amount of blood products (>40 units), and *Candida spp* colonization or infection within 3 months of transplantation. Anti-candida prophylaxis should be considered for patients with these risk factors after liver transplantation.

Aspergillosis is the second most common invasive fungal infections in liver transplant recipients, with an incidence of 11%. Risk factors for invasive aspergillosis in liver transplant recipients are retransplantation, renal failure requiring renal replacement therapy, fulminant hepatic failure as the indication for transplant, and intra-abdominal or thoracic re-exploration within the first month after transplantation. Invasive aspergillosis has the highest mortality in liver transplant recipients compared to other SOT recipients.

Infections After Pancreas and Kidney-Pancreas Transplantation

Kidney-pancreas and pancreas transplant recipients are particularly at risk for surgical-related infections. In general, pancreas transplants are drained into the intestine (called enteric drainage) or the bladder (bladder drainage). The site of drainage has important implications for infectious complications. Enteric drainage poses a risk of abdominal and graft infections, whereas bladder drainage poses a high risk for urinary tract infections and cystitis. Several factors predispose pancreas and kidney-pancreas transplant recipients to infections. First, an individual's diabetes mellitus might be complicated by vascular insufficiency that leads to poor vascular flow and impaired wound healing after transplant. Second, renal failure pre-transplant is a risk factor for infection post-transplant. Third, during transplant, spillage from the contaminated donor duodenum, which is used in the anastomosis between the pancreatic graft and either the intestine or bladder, can contaminate the abdominal cavity. Finally, anastomotic leaks can lead to intra-abdominal infection.

Surgical wound infections occur in 7% to 35% of pancreas transplant recipients and are more common after kidney-pancreas transplantation than kidney transplant alone. Similarly to kidney transplantation, superficial wound infections after kidney-pancreas transplantation are often caused by Gram–positive cocci. Deep wound infections are usually associated with intra- abdominal infections and involve polymicrobial bacteria and *Candida spp* in approximately 50% of the cases.

Intra-abdominal infection is among the most serious complications after pancreas transplant, occurring in 5% to 10% of patients. It is associated with graft loss and can be life-threatening. Sources of intra-abdominal infection include spillage from the donor duodenum; duodenal leaks associated with enteric drainage, and graft inflammation or pancreatitis. The risk factors include donor age, obesity, and recipient's need for peritoneal dialysis and duration of dialysis pre-transplant. Intra-abdominal infections are classified into two broad categories: the life-threatening generalized peritonitis with soilage of the abdominal cavity and localized intra-abdominal abscesses. Both infections are caused by polymicrobial bacteria and yeasts in more than 50% of the cases. The management of the generalized peritonitis requires an emergent exploratory laparotomy to determine and repair the source of the infection and administration of broad spectrum antibacterial and antifungal agents. The management of the localized abscess requires adequate drainage and antimicrobial agents that are directed toward the organisms recovered. Etiology of intra-abdominal abscess is divided into monomicrobial, polymicrobial, and fungal infections. About 50% of the intra-abdominal infections are monomicrobial and caused by *Enterococcus spp.*, *Eschericha coli*, *Klebsiella spp.*, and *Pseudomonas spp.* Extended spectrum β-lactamases-producing and carbapenem ase producing-resistant Gram–negative rods have recently been reported. Polymicrobial and fungal infections are associated with a higher mortality rate. Fungal infection can lead to iliac artery mycotic aneurysm that might rupture. In general, intra-abdominal infection is associated with a poor graft survival at 1 year, a high rate of graft removal of 50%, and a mortality rate of 6% to 20%.

Urinary tract infections are very common after pancreas transplant, and 10% to 20% of these infections are associated with recurrence. Risk factors for UTI in pancreas transplant recipients are related to neurogenic bladder as a complication of diabetes mellitus, alkalinization of the urine from bicarbonate in the pancreatic secretions among patients with bladder drainage, indwelling Foley catheters, and contamination from the donor's duodenum. The most common isolated organisms include *Enterococcus spp*, *Candida spp*, and *Pseudomonas spp* during this period.

Bacteremias are common within the first 3 weeks after pancreas transplant, especially among patients with enteric drainage. In one study, 26% of pancreatic transplant patients with enteric drainage developed bacteremia, and 17% of these are recurrent. Bacteremia co-exists with a site of infection in 69% of cases, including abdominal, vascular catheter, and urinary tract. Overall, bacteremia is associated with a higher mortality and graft loss, as well as higher rate of rejection.

BK virus-associated nephropathy has been described in simultaneous kidney-pancreas (SPK) transplant recipients, with an incidence ranging from 3% to 6%. The average onset of disease is approximately 1 year post-transplantation. Pancreas graft involvement of BK virus has not been described.

Infections After Intestine or Multivisceral Transplant

Infection is the most important cause of morbidity and mortality among recipients of small intestine and multivisceral transplant. Multivisceral transplant includes the stomach, duodenum, pancreas, small intestine, and liver. In general, multivisceral transplant is associated with the highest risk of infections. Bacteria are by far the most important pathogen, and bacterial sepsis accounted for 46% of deaths among intestinal transplant patients. Multiple factors predispose patients to infection. First, the intestinal tract allograft is an immunogenic organ—more so than other intra-abdominal organs—and requires intensive immunosuppressive therapy. Second, indwelling central venous catheters for total parenteral nutrition (TPN) support are generally required for at least a year after transplant. This serves as the source for major bloodstream infection after transplant. Third, transplant procedure is long and extensive, and requirement for re-operation is high. Complications related to the surgical procedure include post-operative hemorrhage, vascular leaks or obstructions, biliary leaks or obstruction, intestinal perforation, and vascular complications such as arterial thrombosis with subsequent graft ischemia and necrosis. These complications might lead to peritonitis, intra-abdominal abscess, and wound dehiscence with evisceration. In addition, the presence of stomata and the problem with insufficient quantity for primary abdominal wall closure might also lead to wound infection. Finally, bacterial overgrowth and translocation during the early post-transplant period arising from ischemia and reperfusion injury or from episodes of rejection or infectious colitis might also lead to intra-abdominal abscess, peritonitis, and bacteremia.

In general, the rates of infections associated with intestinal transplantation are higher than those reported with other intra-abdominal organ transplant, and bacteremia is predominant. In one study, 97% of patients were infected after transplant. Blood is the most common site of infection (41%), followed by lungs (18%), intra-abdominal (16%), surgical wound (11%), and urine (8%). Bacteremia occurs in more than 60% of patients after intestinal transplant and results from vascular catheter/TPN or translocation of the organisms from the GI tract; in approximately 35% of the cases, the source of the infection cannot be determined. Bloodstream infection is caused by polymicrobial organisms in approximately 50% of the cases. The most common organisms associated with bacteremia were *Enteroccocus spp* and *Staphylococcus spp*. A 10-year review of the bloodstream infection from 2000 to 2009 among intestinal transplant patients showed that bacteremia resulting from Gram–positive bacteria decreased from 54% in 2000 to 2003 to 44% in 2007 to 2009. Bacteremia caused by Gram–negative bacteria, on the other hand, increased from 22% in 2000 to 2003 to 43% in 2007 to 2009 ($p = 0.02$). *Candida spp.* and anaerobic bacteria accounted for 11% and 9% of bloodstream infections, respectively, the rates of which did not significantly change over time. The most dramatic increases were noted for *Serratia spp.* (0% to 6.2% in 2000–2003 and 2007–2009, respectively; $p = 0.02$) and *E. coli* (2% to 7%, respectively; $p = 0.05$). The repetitive courses of antibiotics given before and after transplant might provide the selective pressure for emergence of MDR bacteria and yeast organisms.

Intra-abdominal infections, presented as diffuse peritonitis, intra-abddominal abscess and infected fluid collections, are also important infections after intestinal transplant. *Staphylococcus spp.*, *Enterococcus spp.*, *Pseudomona aeruginosa* and members of the *Enterobacteriaceae* group are the most common causative agents. Diffuse peritonitis is associated with a mortality of as high as 50%.

Conclusion

Infections after organ transplantation carry a high morbidity and mortality rate. A detailed understanding of immunosuppression, surgical techniques, and timeline of infections after organ transplantation is essential for effective prevention, timely recognition, and treatment of these infections. The epidemiology of infections is likely to continue to evolve, as advances in immunosuppressive therapy and diagnostic and antimicrobial agents are opening doors for the recognition for rarer disease.

Selected Reference

Fishman JA. Infection in solid-organ transplant recipients. *N Engl J Med* 2007;357(25):2601–2614.

Chapter 10

General Management of Patients in Intensive Care Unit

Faraaz Shah and Sachin Yende

Critically ill patients who are being considered for transplant or who have recently undergone abdominal organ transplantation present unique challenges in providing care. However, the common preventative strategies in the intensive care unit remain equally important. This chapter addresses general principles of management of critically ill patients and highlights important additional considerations in transplant patients. We will focus on:

1. Bed elevation to prevent healthcare-associated pneumonia
2. Preventative strategies against venous thromboembolism
3. Preventative strategies against stress ulcer prophylaxis
4. Paired sedation weaning and spontaneous breathing trials

Elevation of the Head of the Bed

Health care-associated pneumonia (HCAP) is the leading cause of infectious deaths among patients hospitalized in intensive care units (ICUs). In a recent cohort study examining nosocomial infections in ICUs, pneumonia was the underlying cause in more than two-thirds of cases. Patients who develop an episode of nosocomial pneumonia experience an increased length of hospital stay by an average of 7 to 9 days and increased resource consumption and costs per hospitalization. The mortality rate among patients who develop nosocomial pneumonia is estimated to be 20% to 50% higher than in patients who do not develop nosocomial pneumonia.

A particular concern in the ICU is ventilator-associated pneumonia (VAP), defined as pneumonia that develops more than 48 hours after initiation of mechanical ventilation. Similarly to nosocomial pneumonia, VAP is associated with high mortality and approximately 20% to 30% of patients will die during their hospital course. It is unclear whether high mortality results from the pneumonia itself or because VAP occurs in patients who are sick and have multiple-organ dysfunction. The attributable mortality of VAP has been debated extensively, and two recent studies examining large databases of ICU patients have estimated an attributable mortality of 7% to 10%. The increased prevalence of resistant organisms in VAP, such as *Pseudomonas aeruginosa* and methicillin-resistant *Staphylococcus auereus*, and the associated difficulty in treating these organisms, combined with the increase in hospital stays and resource utilization, highlight the importance of implementing strategies to reduce their incidence.

Risk factors for Health Care-Associated Pneumonia

Table 10.1 describes risk factors for HCAP in critically ill patients. The most significant risk factor in the ICU is mechanical ventilation. Although the risk of HCAP in patients with liver disease or transplantation has not been studied extensively, these patients are likely to be at an increased risk for several reasons.

First, patients who undergo transplant often require mechanical ventilation prior to transplant because of infection, encephalopathy, or gastrointestinal (GI) bleeding, and in the immediate post-operative period.

Second, patients with underlying liver disease have impaired immune response. Immunosuppressive medications used after transplantation may impair cell-mediated immunity. Intubation leaves patients unable to utilize their innate defenses against developing pneumonia, including the cough reflex and the mucociliary clearance of lower respiratory secretions.

Third, altered mental status caused by hepatic encephalopathy may also increase risk of aspiration and subsequently of pneumonia, akin to higher risk of pneumonia reported in prior studies in patients with neurological conditions (odds ratio [OR] = 3.4).

Fourth, repeated episodes of intubation for procedures, such as upper GI hemorrhage, may injure the respiratory tract and increase susceptibility to infection.

Finally, transplant patients often have higher burden of chronic diseases, which are associated with higher risk of pneumonia, such as respiratory disease (OR = 2.8) and cardiac disease (OR = 2.3).

Preventative Strategies

Prevention of nosocomial pneumonia and VAP is essential in newly transplanted patients, as infections in newly transplanted patients are a significant cause of increased morbidity and mortality. Overall infection rates as high as 33% to 66% following liver transplant have been reported, and in the first month, bacterial infections tend to predominate. Common sites of infection are surgical

Table 10.1 Risk Factors for Nosocomial Pneumonia
Mechanical ventilation
Pre-existing heart disease
Central nervous system impairment
Male gender
Witnessed aspiration
Trauma
Burns

site, lungs, urinary tract, and catheter insertion sites, with a higher incidence of Gram–negative bacteria, including *Pseudomonas aueruginosa*. Low pre-operative albumin, need for hemodialysis, and prolonged ICU stays increase this risk of infection in orthotopic liver transplant recipients.

Several preventative strategies have been examined to reduce the risk of HCAP, including oropharyngeal decontamination, probiotics, silver-coated endotracheal tubes, closed-circuit suction tubes, and patient positioning. Of these strategies, elevation of the head end of the patient bed in mechanically ventilated patients has been studied most extensively. Elevation of the head of the bed is easy to implement without additional cost and has few, if any, adverse effects.

The Center for Disease Control recommends that ventilated patients should ideally be placed in the semi-recumbent position with the head of the bed elevated at an inclination of 30 to 45 degrees. Several randomized controlled trials have demonstrated that maintaining patients in the semi-recumbent position decreases the incidence of VAP. In a randomized controlled trial by Drakulovic et al. the incidence of VAP was 34% among patients maintained in a supine position and 8% ($p = 0.003$) in those maintained in the semi-recumbent position. Similarly, confirmed cases of VAP were 23% and 5%, respectively ($p = 0.018$).

A study reported that compared to supine position, elevated head position reduced the incidence of pneumonia by 50% (OR = 0.47, 95 % CI = 0.27–0.82). However, these effects were greatly reduced when bed elevation was not consistently maintained. Trends toward improved survival and decreased hospital stay, which did not approach statistical significance, were also noted in this meta-analysis. This protective effect is believed to result from decreased aspiration of gastric contents and ensuing colonization of the respiratory tract with the head of the bed elevated compared to in the supine position.

Despite these benefits, elevating the head of the bed is still not consistently achieved, in part because of constraints with other aspects of patient and nursing care. Potential strategies to improve compliance include inclusion in ventilator-bundles and admission order sets, where they may be paired with other effective measures against VAP. Education of nursing staff and respiratory therapists to work collaboratively and to emphasize the importance of this simple maneuver may improve compliance. Routine audits to assess compliance with the intervention in a prominent place in the ICUs to encourage change and motivate staff may also be considered.

Prone positioning has also been evaluated as a potential measure to decrease incidence of VAP. Although prone positioning does improve oxygenation in patients with acute lung injury, it does not change the risk of developing nosocomial pneumonia nor does it decrease associated mortality.

Thromboembolism Prophylaxis

Critically ill patients are at an increased risk of thromboembolism, and appropriate prophylaxis in the post-transplant patient is essential. However, compliance within ICUs varies, with some rates reported as low as 33%.

Although the incidence of venous thromboembolism (VTE) in the general population is only 0.2% to 0.3%, incidences rises to 10% to 25% among those admitted to the hospital. Development of VTE is believed to evolve from abnormalities in endothelial injury, venous stasis, and hypercoaguability. Critically ill transplant recipients carry a number of risk factors that place them at high risk (see Table 10.2).

However, these patients are also at high risk of bleeding. For example, patients with liver disease or those in the immediate post-transplant period have coagulopathy and complications related to portal venous hypertension, which may increase the risk of bleeding. Thus, VTE prophylaxis is often not instituted. Rates of VTE in cirrhotic patients are typically lower than in the general population, but patients will still develop deep vein and portal vein thromboses. An elevated INR level is not reflective of a protected state against VTE, and patients may still develop clots. This may result in part from defective synthesis of Protein C and S and antithrombin III in end-stage cirrhosis. Prophylaxis can be used carefully in selected individuals based on their risk for bleeding or recent bleeding events. Notably, risk factors associated with VTE in cirrhotic patients, such as increased MELD scores, worse Child's class, and higher alpha-fetoprotein levels are also risk factors for GI bleeding. Patients with concomitant cirrhosis and hepatic malignancy have a four- to seven-fold increase in VTE compared to those who do not, and VTE prophylaxis should be strongly considered for these patients. Patients who are candidates for small bowel transplant or who have undergone small bowel transplantation have co-existing hypercoagulable states, such as protein C and protein S deficiency. Thus, these patients may be at high-risk for VTE.

Non-Pharmacological Measures to Prevent Venous Thromboembolism

Non-pharmacological methods against VTE are available, although pharmacological methods are preferred if there is no contraindication. Graduated compression stockings aim to prevent the pooling of blood in the lower extremities and prevent the development of venous clots. When appropriately used, compression stockings have been shown to decrease the rate of deep vein thrombosis. Fitting patients with appropriately sized compression stockings can be challenging, and if the stockings are not properly fitted, then the risk of VTE is actually increased.

Table 10.2 Risk Factors for Development of Venous Thromboembolism
Age greater than 75 years
Cancer
Acute infection
Chronic respiratory abnormalities
Confinement
Central venous catheters
Heart failure

Pneumatic compression stockings applied to the lower extremities similarly operate by intermittently inflating and squeezing blood through the venous system to reduce the risk of venous stasis. Use of pneumatic compression stockings in medical and surgical ICUs have shown benefit in reducing the risk of VTE but are considered less effective when compared to low-molecular-weight heparins (LMWHs). A Cochrane review meta-analysis demonstrated that the addition of pneumatic compression stockings to usual prophylaxis reduced the incidence of post-operative pulmonary embolism in cardiac surgery patients to 1.5% compared to 4% with subcutaneous heparin alone, a relative reduction of 62%.

Pharmacological Interventions to Prevent Venous Thromboembolism

Unfractionated heparin is most commonly used for prophylaxis against VTE. Both naturally derived unfractionated heparin (UFH) and LMWHs, containing only short-chain heparins, have been show to decrease the incidence of clinically detected VTE compared to placebo. Head-to-head trials comparing UFH and LMWHs have demonstrated similar rates of prevention and similar rates of major bleeding. Many trials have also demonstrated slightly improved prevention with LMWHs, such as enoxaparin, particularly in patients with underlying malignancy. Low-molecular-weight heparins are often used with caution in patients with renal dysfunction for concerns of accumulation.

Vitamin K antagonists such as warfarin are used in treatment of VTE and provide protection against the development of future thromboembolism. Vitamin K antagonists, however, are not often used as primary prevention in the immediate post-operative period.

Newer options include direct thrombin inhibitors such as dabigatran, which have been shown to be non-inferior to slightly worse in preventing VTE compared to LMWHs in recent clinical trials. Fondaparinux, a synthetic Factor Xa inhibitor, has also been approved for use of prevention of DVT/PE in surgical patients and in the medically ill. Direct Factor Xa inhibitors apixaban and rivaroxaban are also emerging as new alternatives for treatment and prevention of VTE, demonstrating superior results when compared to lovenox in preventing VTE in patients who are undergoing hip arthroplasties without an increase in major bleeding.

Standard VTE prophylaxis, using compression stockings and pneumatic compression devices, should be used in all patients. Additionally, UFH can be used carefully in those without recent bleeding and without significant coagulopathy. Additionally, LMWHs have been proven to be a safe option for treatment of portal vein thrombosis in patients with cirrhosis and portal vein thrombosis and would be an acceptable option in those at high risk for VTE, such as those with malignancy.

Stress Ulcer Prophylaxis

Nosocomial bleeding of the GI tract, particularly bleeding of the upper GI tract, has been associated with increased morbidity and mortality in patients admitted to a hospital. Stress-related mucosal injury can occur in ICU patients within the first few days of ICU admission. The most important risk factors for the development of GI bleeding are coagulopathy and need for mechanical ventilation. Other risk factors include history of GI bleeding, hypotension, and multi-organ system dysfunction. Most of these risk factors are common prior to and in the immediate post-operative period after transplant. Gastrointestinal bleeding following liver transplant increases mortality following transplant and has been associated with increased re-exploration surgery. Clinically significant bleeding following liver transplant occurs more frequently in the first few months following transplant. An early study identified gastric ulcers as the most common cause, followed by enteritis and portal hypertensive bleeding. Additionally small bowel patients may bleed from anastomotic sites.

Preventative measures focus on gastric acid suppression. Early trials of acid suppression used antacids, sucralfates, and H2 blockers and reported benefit in decreasing the incidence of both clinically significant and life-threatening GI bleeding. With reductions in clinically detected bleeding up to 40% in early trials using H2 blockers, many clinical practice guidelines endorse GI prophylaxis in mechanically ventilated patients and in the critically ill.

Proton pump inhibitors (PPIs), which increase gastric pH by antagonistic effects on H+/K+ ATPases, are now commonly used as prophylactic measures against GI bleeding, even beyond the critical care setting. Proton pump inhibitors are more potent than H2 blockers in increasing gastric pH in critically ill patients; however, no study has shown improved efficacy with PPI to prevent GI bleeding. Current guidelines advocate the use of GI prophylaxis in the critically ill; however, follow-up studies have failed to show the same benefit of routine gastric acid suppression in decreasing mortality from GI bleeding, while demonstrating an association with increased incidence of infection. More recent observational studies have also reported decreased incidence of stress ulcer and GI bleeding compared to earlier trials, as low as 1% to 2% of critically ill patients. The reasons behind these improved outcomes are unknown but may include more aggressive early resuscitation of patients and early introduction of enteral feeds; the latter has been known to increase gastric pH and may help prevent mucosal ulcerations. Inclusion of patients who are not high risk for bleeding in these studies may contribute lower rates of bleeding.

Long-term use of PPIs has been associated with increased risk of community-acquired pneumonia, as well as HCAP and Clostridium difficile infection. The increased risk of infection is believed to be related to the alteration of gastric mucosal flora with acid suppressive medication and ensuing bacterial overgrowth.

This risk of infection is an important consideration before institution of stress ulcer prophylaxis in abdominal organ transplant patients who will have impaired immunity prior to surgery and will be immunosuppressed following their transplant. For patients with an average risk of bleeding, routine prophylaxis with H2 blockers will help reduce the risk of clinically significant bleeding without the increased risk of infections. Proton pump inhibitors can be considered when the risk of GI bleeding outweighs the potential risk of infection, including patients who have underlying peptic ulcer disease or are at high risk for bleeding.

Daily Sedation Interruption Trials

Patients with liver or renal disease often require sedation or use of opioids prior to transplantation or during the immediate post-operative period because of use of mechanical ventilation. Sedatives are commonly used to increase comfort and synchronization while intubated; however, these same medications may increase delirium and cause over-sedation. Thus efforts should be undertaken to achieve an appropriate balance between minimizing use of sedatives and pain medications and maintaining comfort.

In patients with liver disease, use of sedatives should be carefully titrated because hepatic dysfunction impairs clearance and alters the pharmacokinetics of these drugs. Alterations in plasma protein binding, biliary excretion, enterohepatic circulation, and changes in renal clearance caused by concomitant renal disease may also alter metabolism of intravenously administered drugs and necessitate close monitoring. Further, the clinical effects may vary in these patients, independent of drug bio-availability, because of alterations in cerebral drug receptors resulting in variable sensitivity to opioids and sedatives. In general, lowest doses of short-acting sedatives and opioids should be used.

Daily Sedation Interruption

A landmark 2 x 2 factorial randomized controlled trial involving 128 adult patients was conducted to assess the efficacy of daily sedation interruption strategies and compared propofol and midazolam for sedation in patients receiving mechanical ventilation. Ventilated patients who had stable sedative requirements were randomized to spontaneous awakening trials in the intervention group, where the sedative infusions were interrupted on a daily basis until the patients were awake. In the control group, the infusions were interrupted only at the discretion of the clinicians. Patients in the intervention group who developed signs of distress or agitation within 4 hours as assessed by a physician were considered to have failed, and sedation was resumed, but those who did not develop distress simply kept off of sedation. The median duration of mechanical ventilation was 4.9 days in the intervention group versus 7.3 days in the control group, and the median lengths of stay in the ICU were 6.4 days and 9.9 days, respectively. Use of sedatives was less in the intervention group. The beneficial effects of sedation interruption in this study occurred because it may have prevented accumulation of the drug and its metabolites, an important consideration in patients with liver disease.

Concerns were raised that spontaneous awakening trials may increase the risk of late emotional sequelae following ICU hospitalization and potentially increase the risk of ICU complications including VAP, barotrauma, thromboembolic disease, and GI hemorrhage. Subsequent studies have demonstrated that spontaneous awakening trials do not increase the risk of ICU complications during hospitalization or the risk of post-traumatic stress disorder during subsequent months.

Pairing Spontaneous Breathing Trials

Because initiation of the spontaneous breathing trials (SBTs) requires discontinuation or reduction of sedative and analgesic medications, subsequent trials paired sedation weaning protocols with SBTs and demonstrated improved outcomes. The Awakening and Breathing Controlled trial randomly assigned 336 mechanically ventilated critically ill patients to receive either protocolized paired spontaneous awakening and SBTs or usual care coupled with SBTs. Patients in the intervention group were evaluated daily for safety of spontaneous awakening trials and underwent interruptions in sedatives and analgesics. Those who failed were restarted at one-half the previous sedative dose and titrated back up, and those who passed were advanced to the SBT protocol. Patients who took spontaneous breaths and maintained an arterial oxygen saturation above 88% on lower oxygen and lower positive end-expiratory pressure requirements underwent SBT with reduced ventilatory support, such as breathing through either a T-tube circuit or on low settings of continuous positive airway pressure. Patients who developed agitation, tachycardia, tachypnea, or respiratory failure on SBTs were considered to have failed them. Patients who passed a SBT were considered for extubation.[5] After SI/SBT, if patients were not extubated, then they were restarted on half of the original dose of sedative medications.

The patients in the protocolized to SI/SBT group had greater ventilator-free time over 28 days (mean difference of 3.1 days, 95% CI 0.7–5.6 days), earlier discharge from the ICU (9.1 days vs. 12.9 days compared to controls), and higher 1-year survival (hazard ratio [HR] = 0.68, 95% CI 0.50–0.92).

Subsequent studies confirmed these findings and continued to demonstrate that protocolized SBT paired with SI were effective in decreasing the time spent on mechanical ventilation and the overall risk of death. The rates of self-extubation are slightly higher in patients undergoing paired sedation and awakening trials compared to those who do not; however, the rates of reintubation are similar.

An alternative approach that is emerging is an opioid-only approach for sedation while on mechanical ventilation. A recent single-center, randomized controlled study compared protocols of continuous sedation using propofol and midazolam with daily SI to an experimental protocol with as needed boluses of morphine and found that patients in the opioid-only group had 4.2 fewer days on mechanical ventilation and 9.7 fewer days in the ICU. Patients randomized to opioid-only arm experienced higher rates of agitation. An important limitation of this trial was that it increased nursing burden. For example, the study included caregivers to reassure patients who were agitated, and nurse–patient ratio was 1:1. Finally, despite these interventions, some patients in the analgesic group did require sedation. This study highlights the potential for an alternative strategy that minimizes exposure to sedating medications, including benzodiazepines.

This approach may be an attractive option for critically ill transplant patients with hepatic dysfunction.

Sedation interruption also allows for patients to participate in earlier physical and occupational rehabilitation therapy. Pairing sedation weaning with physical therapy in which patients performed active range of motion as tolerated while mechanically ventilated has been shown to also help decrease the time to functional independence and improve recovery following critical illness. Paired sedation weaning and spontaneous breathing trials should thus be initiated soon after transplantation to help improve outcomes and reduce ICU stays.

Selected References

Cook DJ & Crowther MA. Thromboprophylaxis in the intensive care unit: focus on medical-surgical patients. *Crit Care Med*. 2010;38(2 Suppl):S76–S82.

Dellinger RP, Levy MM, Carlet JM, et al. International Surviving Sepsis Campaign Guidelines Committee.international guidelines for management of severe sepsis and septic shock. *Crit Care Med*. 2008;36(1):296–327.

Drakulovic MB, Torres A, Bauer TT, et al. Supine body positioning as a risk factor for nosocomial pneumonia in mechanically ventilated patients: A randomized trial. *Lancet*. 1999;354(9193):1851–1858.

Girard TD, Kress JP, Fuchs BD, Thomason JW, et al. Efficacy and safety of a paired sedation and ventilator weaning protocol for mechanically ventilated patients in intensive care (Awakening and Breathing Controlled trial): a randomised controlled trial. *Lancet*. 2008;371(9607):126–134.

Marik PE, Vasu T, Hirani A, & Pachinburavan M. Stress ulcer prophylaxis in the new millennium: a systematic review and meta-analysis. *Crit Care Med*. 2010;38(11):2222–2228.

Chapter 11

Nursing Considerations

Susan DeRubis, Kate Foryte, Kristy Bayer, and Tracy Grogan

High-quality nursing care is an essential component of transplantation success. Transplant procedures are often lengthy, placing a high degree of physiological stress on the patient. It is important that the nurse in the intensive care unit (ICU) receiving the patient be organized and ready to perform many simultaneous tasks. Prior to the arrival of the patient from the operating room, (OR), it is the responsibility of the bedside nurse to ensure that the bed space is efficiently configured and that all necessary equipment is ready. Figure 11.1 illustrates the typical ICU room ready for the transplanted patient.

Note the following equipment starting from the left and moving clockwise around the room:
- Multiple IV pumps to manage multiple infusions
  - Cardiac drips
  - Sedation
  - Analgesia
  - IV fluids
- Pressure infusing saline flush bags
- Transducer holder
- Cardiac monitor mounted on the top of the tower
- Continuous cardiac output monitor located at the head of the bed
- Ventilator

Most transplant patients arrive with the following central lines: a multilumen pulmonary artery catheter as a component of a large bore right internal jugular introducer, a secondary introducer (usually left internal jugular), and two arterial catheters. In addition, the patient may arrive with an internal Doppler catheter that provides an auditory signal of vessel patency, and the monitoring device (not pictured) would be mounted on a pole to the left of the patient. Meticulous organization allows for the smooth and safe transition from the OR to ICU setting.

A team of ICU providers is present as the patient arrives from the OR, including nurses, critical care physicians, respiratory therapists, and patient care technicians. Once the patient arrives, safe hand-off reporting occurs between the surgical/anesthesia team and the bedside nurse. This report describes the medical/surgical history, major clinical events during and at the end of surgery, recent lab values, fluid balance, the need for vasoactive medications during the case,

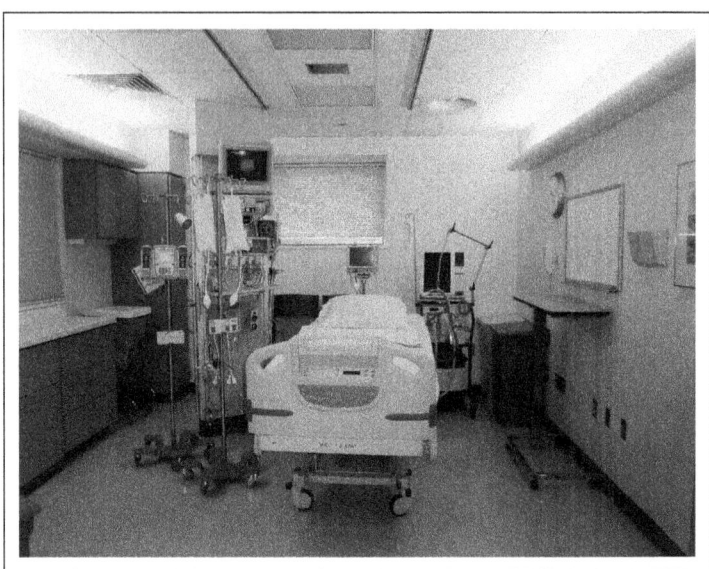

Figure 11.1. ICU room prior to admission of newly transplanted patient.

other medications administered, and current state of anesthesia and pain control. The patient is connected to the monitor, the endotracheal tube is secured and ventilator settings checked. A primary assessment of airway, breathing, and circulation is completed. Blood specimens are drawn for an initial set of values that may include arterial and venous blood gases, electrolytes, complete blood count with differential and platelets, calcium, magnesium, phosphorous, BUN, creatinine, liver function tests, and coagulation studies. Invasive monitoring devices are assessed for proper waveforms and calibrated. A chest X-ray provides confirmation of endotracheal tube and invasive line placement as well as radiographic assessment for pulmonary complications. Body temperature is obtained and measures to achieve/maintain normothermia are implemented. Tubes and drains are evaluated for drainage quantity, color, and viscosity, as illustrated in Figure 11.2. Incisions may vary in size and shape depending on the type of organ transplant performed and complications encountered during surgery. Incision sites may be closed through all layers or occasionally closed at the skin layer only and secured with either staples or sutures. At times, the abdomen may be left open with internal mesh or with a wound vacuum dressing to accommodate planned future surgeries. Most transplant patients have drains postoperatively but the number and type of drains placed vary with the surgery type and the surgeon's preference. Figure 11.2 illustrates the postoperative abdomen of a liver transplant patient. The inverted Y or Mercedes incision is typical. To the right side of the patient are two Jackson–Pratt (JP) drains. When

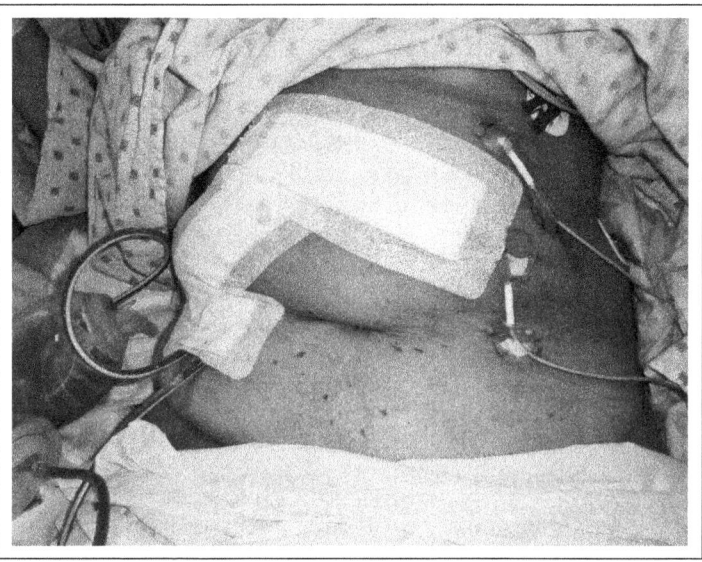

Figure 11.2. Tubes and drains associated with postoperative abdominal transplant.

the patient arrives in the ICU, the transplant surgeon reviews with the nurses the exact location of each drain. In general, at least two drains are placed, one located behind the liver near the inferior vena cava anastomosis and the second placed near the hilum to assess for biliary duct leakage. When a drain is placed to assess for biliary leakage, a small amount of bilious drainage is expected. In some cases, a biliary drain may be placed in the right upper quadrant of the abdomen. When present, the nurse inspects this drain for changes in quantity and quality of bile produced. During the immediate postoperative period, it is not unusual to see dark brown drainage if Surgicel® has been used during the case. Lastly, the left side of the abdomen shows two internal Doppler catheters. Vessel patency is monitored continuously by an auditory signal. It is important that the nurse is attentive to subtle changes in the drainage and report these changes to the surgical team immediately.

If the patient is hemodynamically unstable on arrival to the unit, the nurses and physicians work collaboratively at the bedside to assess and correct any immediate problems. Fluid and/or blood products may be ordered and administered rapidly along with frequent titrations of vasoactive medications. Rarely, an emergent bedside procedure may be required in which the nurses assist.

Once the initial block of assessments is complete and cardiopulmonary stability is achieved, the post-operative orders must be diligently reviewed. At minimum, these orders should include:

• Maintenance IV fluid, including type and rate

- Sedation orders with titration and weaning parameters
- Analgesia orders
- Routine and serial labwork
- DVT prophylaxis
- Ventilator orders with weaning parameters
- Blood glucose checks with coverage parameters
- ICU nursing protocol orders such as electrolyte replacement
- Fluid boluses and/or blood product orders
- Vasoactive drips with titration parameters
- Foley catheter

Finally, the nurse must ensure that routine medications are ordered and administered—especially anti-rejection agents—paying particular attention to when the first dose is due. The nurse also ensures antibiotics, antivirals, antifungals, stress ulcer prophylaxis, antihypertensives, and antiemetics are ordered.

A complete head-to-toe assessment (Table 11.1) follows, which may be combined with bathing to prepare the patient for family visitation. During this assessment, all skin surfaces are inspected for areas of breakdown, redness, or pallor. The postoperative patient baseline assessment is established, from which future changes will be evaluated. Table 11.2 highlights common postoperative problems. The bedside nurse monitors for subtle changes that could become catastrophic if not recognized early.

An often overlooked but large part of the care provided by the bedside nurse involves family support. The families of transplant patients are under incredible stress. The stressors are multifactorial: the fear and anxiety of living with someone with a chronic, debilitating, life-threatening disease; financial stress; isolation and the added burden of shouldering a larger portion of family responsibilities. The bedside nurse is the constant contact person and conduit of vital information for families. The information that must be processed by families is often complex and overwhelming, requiring the bedside nurse to refine skills in providing information multiple times in small, understandable pieces. The nurse is often the only one available to listen to the concerns of the family and advocate for their needs. Often, family frustration is released upon the bedside nurse who must be skilled in diffusing potentially volatile situations and finding a satisfactory resolution. The transplant nurse must not only be highly skilled clinically, but must possess exemplary psychosocial skills. The transplant nurse is never more than a few steps away from the patient during the immediate postoperative period. Ultimately, recovery may be directly related to the skill level of the bedside nurse and his/her ability to recognize and react appropriately to changes.

Table 11.1 Nursing Head-to-Toe Assessment Parameters of the Immediate Postoperative Abdominal Transplant Patient

Neurological	Level of sedation and subsequent waking pattern, PERRLA, pain assessment.
Cardiovascular	Hemodynamic parameters: BP, CO, PA, CVP, PPV, lab values, metabolic imbalances that could lead to cardiac dysfunction/arrhythmias, signs and symptoms of bleeding, Doppler monitoring of grafted vessels, pulses (presence and quality), edema.
Respiratory	Ventilator settings and weaning parameters, lung sounds, secretions (amount, color, consistency), implement VAP prevention measures, continuous pulse oximeter monitoring, SVO2 monitoring.
Gastrointestinal	Assessment of all tubes/drains, which may include nasogastric tube, nasoduodenal feeding tube, gastric-jejunal tube, Jackson–Pratt drains, T-tube, ostomies, and fistula drainage sites. Each tube and/or drain is assessed for patency, drainage color, quantity, viscosity, signs of bleeding, or bile leakage. The incision site is noted for signs of dehiscence, drainage, redness, edema, or purulence. Bowel sounds and flatus are monitored for return of gut motility.
Genitourinary	Urinary catheter type noted, urine quality—color, consistency, sediment, odor, hourly urine output. Closely monitor, coordinate with IV fluid replacement if ordered.
Skin	Open skin areas and pressure injuries noted. Appropriate skin care referrals obtained.
Infectious Disease	Assess for potential areas of infection, invasive line insertion sites; apply dressings following sterile technique; wash perineal area with soap and water; clean and apply dressing to incisional site; assess for areas of redness, warmth, and purulent drainage; monitor lab values.
Endocrine	Monitor blood glucose levels and provide correction coverage as ordered.

Table 11.2 Bedside Nurse Monitoring of Postoperative Transplant Complications

Neurological	Titration of sedation to facilitate assessment of awakening from general anesthesia, ability to follow commands, effect of sedation on VS, readiness for ventilator weaning, and extubation. Recognition of inability to awaken from sedation that may lead to further testing (CT scan, EEG). Assess level of pain, and medicate as ordered. Consistently observe for mental status changes that may be indicators of issues such as: CO_2 retention, antirejection toxicity, ICU psychosis, withdrawal from previous psychiatric meds, etc.
Cardio vascular	Closely monitor hemodynamic parameters (CO, BP, PPV, CVP, PA pressures, sVO2, body temp, etc.), which may be the first indicators of hemorrhage/volume depletion or early sepsis. Serial labs are meticulously observed for changes in H/H, coagulation factors, and electrolyte imbalances. Electrolyte protocols are used to enable the nurse to correct early imbalances independently. Management of all invasive lines is imperative for patient safety. Nurses in the ICU are responsible for assistance with new line insertion and removing of lines if ordered.
Respiratory	Monitor for readiness for early extubation. Monitor for changes in ventilation status, such as increasing FiO2 and PEEP requirements, changes in lung sounds, and secretions. VAP prevention weighs heavily on the nurse and includes diligent mouth care, elevating the head of the bed, and frequent positioning/mobilization to aid in pulmonary toileting. Management of chest tubes if present.
Gastrointestinal	Frequent assessment of abdominal incisions and drains for changes in drainage amount, color, and consistency. Management of multiple incisions, drains, and the internal Doppler. Assuring GI ulcer prophylaxis and early nutrition is ordered and administered. Careful observation of the abdomen for increasing tenderness, distention, restoration of flatus, and bowel movement. Ostomy care and monitoring of stoma/output.
Renal	Strict hourly I&O, paying attention to changes in quantity and quality of urine produced. Adhere to hourly fluid replacement as ordered. Pay attention to urine output, as it relates to changes in hemodynamic status.
Rejection	Send daily lab work and monitor immune suppression medication levels. Work closely with transplant team with regard to medication dosage changes. Monitor closely for possible signs and symptoms of rejection—that is, changes in lab values, increased jaundice, ascites, changes in ostomy appearance/drainage, and changes in urine output.
Infection	Ensure strict handwashing of all health-care professionals and family members. Meticulous oral hygiene, catheter care, invasive line care (including early removal), bathing with antimicrobial cleansers, and containment of draining body fluids so as not to contaminate incisions and open skin areas. Diligent monitoring of hemodynamic parameters that may indicate early sepsis.
Skin breakdown	Turning and repositioning at least every 2 hours, early mobilization, excellent skin care that includes washing and moisturizing, daily rotation of ET tube, and cushioning of tracheostomies, providing skin inspections for reddened or open areas. Obtain orders for wound-healing ointments when needed.

Chapter 12

Indications for Liver Transplantation

Jana G. Hashash and Kapil B. Chopra

Introduction

Liver transplantation remains to be the only hope for cure and survival in patients with decompensated end-stage liver disease (ESLD), acute/fulminant liver failure, and those with primary hepatic malignancies. Transplanting a new organ not only requires a fit patient and a matching donor but also mandates the presence of a social support system and an experienced multidisciplinary team, consisting of transplant coordinators, hepatologists, liver transplant surgeons, psychiatrists, social workers, as well as critical care physicians. The health-care providers together with the patients and their support system function as a group throughout the pre-transplantation period and as importantly in the post-operative period as well. Currently, liver disease and the need for precious organs are on the rise, surpassing the number of available livers for donation. In this chapter we will present an overview of the criteria for accepting patients to the transplantation list, the indications for liver transplantation, as well as the absolute and relative contraindications for liver transplantation.

Background

The first human liver transplant operation was performed by Dr. Thomas Starzl in 1963. Over the following 20 years, there was evolution in the criteria for listing, surgical techniques, as well as the post-operative care including immunosuppression management, aggressive rehabilitation, and follow-up, increasing the success rates of those transplant operations. Today, the 1-year patient survival after deceased donor liver transplant is approximately 86%; the 5-year survival is 72%; and the 10-year survival is 56%. The 1-year graft survival is approximately 81%, 5-year graft survival is 64%, and 10-year graft survival is 46%. The operation is titled orthotopic liver transplantation because the recipient's damaged liver gets replaced by a healthy donor liver allograft in the same anatomic location. Most transplants include deceased-donor grafts, but because there is a paucity in the number of donors compared to the number of livers needed, live-donor liver transplantations, splitting deceased-donor grafts, and the use of marginal or extended grafts have been performed to increase the availability of organs. Marginal grafts include those livers from older patients and from non-heart-beating donors. Live-donor liver transplantations are slightly riskier than the other operations because of the potential complications they pose on the donor.

Listing Criteria

Model of End-Stage Liver Disease Era

In the past, organs were allocated to patients using the Child-Pugh-Turcotte (CPT) scoring system along with other clinical criteria. The minimal listing criteria for liver transplantation included (1) CPT score $\geq$ 7, (2) ascites, (3) gastrointestinal bleeding secondary to portal hypertension, and (4) spontaneous bacterial peritonitis.

As of February 2002, the Model of End-Stage Liver Disease (MELD) score has been used to assign priority to patients on the liver transplantation wait list. The CPT scoring system assesses the severity of liver disease, whereas the MELD score is an objective scoring system that predicts the short-term mortality of patients with liver cirrhosis. Although, the CPT classification is widely used when evaluating patients with liver cirrhosis; nowadays the MELD score alone is used to stratify patients on the transplant list. Many reasons drove the United Network for Organ Sharing (UNOS) to adapt this change. Such reasons include the subjectivity behind some of the CPT parameters such as determining the presence and degree of ascites and that of hepatic encephalopathy. Also, the CPT scoring system has a "ceiling effect" where patients with an international normalized ratio (INR) of 2.4 received a similar score to those with an INR of 4 or even 9, and those with a total serum bilirubin of 10 mg/dL received the same score as those with a bilirubin level of 3.1 mg/dL. Table 12.1 demonstrates the CPT parameters and scoring system. A score between 5 and 6 signifies a Class A cirrhotic, a score between 7 and 9 is a Class B cirrhotic, whereas a score of 10 and above is a Class C cirrhotic. At least 35% of Class C patients die while waiting on the transplantation list within 1 year, whereas 90% of patients with Class A survive for the next 5 years without a liver transplantation.

The MELD score is an objective calculation based on a patient's serum creatinine, serum total bilirubin, and INR using the following formula (http://www.mayoclinic.org/meld/mayomodel6.html):

$$\text{MELD score} = (0.975 \times \ln(\text{serum creatinine}) + 0.378 \times \ln(\text{serum bilirubin}) + 1.120 \times \ln(\text{INR}) + 0.643) \times 10$$

In patients on hemodyalysis, the serum creatinine is automatically considered as 4.0.

The liver transplantation list uses the MELD score as an indicator of priority for liver allocation. Those patients with a higher MELD score are more ill with a higher

Table 12.1 Child-Pugh-Turcotte

	Points		
	1	2	3
Hepatic Encephalopathy	Absent	Mild	Severe
Enceplopathy	Absent	Mild/Moderate	Severe/ Refractory
Total bilirubin	<2 mg/dL,	2–3 mg/dL	>3 mg/dL
INR	<1.7	1.7–2.3	>2.3
Albumin	>3.5	2.8–3.5	<2.8

INR: international normalized ratio

short-term mortality. Therefore, these patients are higher on the list compared to other candidates with lower MELD scores. The concept of survival benefit-based deceased-donor liver allocation was proposed by Merion et al. wherein allocation of deceased-donor livers to chronic liver failure patients would be improved by prioritizing patients by transplant survival benefit. Patients whose MELD score is less than 15 have a higher survival rate without transplantation. Patients whose score is less than 10 are not listed unless they qualify for exceptions and extra points, as detailed below. Referral for liver transplantation should be made when the survival of those patients is predicted to be less than 95% at 1 year.

Model for End-Stage Liver Disease Exceptions

In certain situations, the MELD score is not reflective of a patient's true clinical status because the short-term mortality of these patients does not directly result from their underlying liver disease. This unfortunately has led to prolonged waiting times and deaths of critically ill patients whose MELD scores were not appropriately reflective of the severity of their overall clinical condition. This prompted UNOS to modify their listing criteria and allow for certain exceptions. Some exceptions qualify for extra points to be added to the native MELD scores of patients bringing these patients higher on the list, whereas other exceptions allow for prioritizing certain patients without a change in the absolute MELD number. Those exceptions included will be described below and are demonstrated in Table 12.2. There appears to be regional variations in the United States with respect to the use of "MELD exceptions" in organ allocation for liver transplantation.

a. Ascites

Ascites is a well-known complication of liver cirrhosis (Fig. 12.1) that is associated with an increased mortality risk. Although the presence of ascites does not automatically add points to patients' MELD scores, patients with refractory ascites or complicated ascites can be prioritized. The criteria for defining refractory or complicated ascites includes massive abdominal distention documented radiographically in addition to the presence of two of the following six criteria:

(1) prior transjugular intrahepatic portosystemic shunt placement;

(2) at least two episodes of spontaneous bacterial peritonitis;

Table 12.2 MELD Exceptions

Ascites (Refractory or severe)
Hepatic encephalopathy
Polycystic liver disease
Gastrointestinal bleeding
Hepatopulmonary syndrome
Portopulmonary syndrome
Budd-Chiari syndrome
Primary hyperoxaluria
Familial amyloid polyneuropathy
Cystic fibrosis
Cholangiocarcinoma
Cholangitis
Unusual tumor
Unusual metabolic disease
Small-for-size syndrome
Hereditary hemorrhagic telengectasia

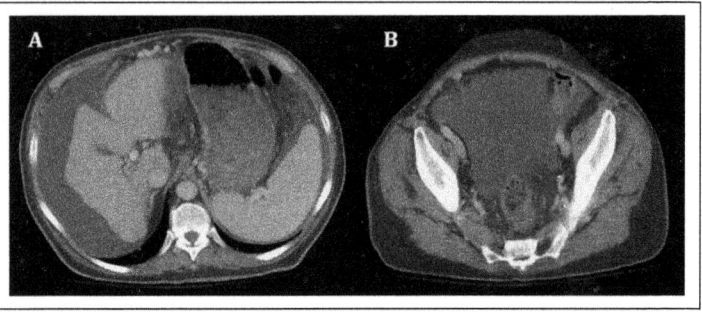

Figure 12.1. **(A)** Perihepatic ascites and **(B)** revealing pelvic ascites in the same patient.

(3) at least three therapeutic abdominal paracenteses in the last 60 days (each removing at least 2 liters);

(4) ascites unresponsive to maximum diuretic therapy consisting of 400 mg of spironolactone daily and 160 mg of furosemide daily;

(5) serum sodium 125 mEq/L or less; or

(6) at least two therapeutic thoracenteses procedures.

b. Portosystemic Encephalopathy

Similarly to ascites, hepatic encephalopathy is a commonly encountered complication of liver cirrhosis, also associated with an increased mortality risk. Patients with hepatic encephalopathy do not get extra MELD points, but if their encephalopathy is severe, then they may be prioritized. Severe encephalopathy includes patients with cerebral edema and high intracranial pressures, those with grade IV encephalopathy who require endotracheal intubation, and those who are profoundly encephalopathic because of large portosystemic shunts.

c. Polycystic Liver Disease

Polycystic liver disease rarely leads to complications of ESLD but usually leads to malnutrition and problems with the cysts themselves, including infection or rupture. Patients with massive polycystic liver disease (total cyst: parenchyma ratio >1), those with severe malnutrition, and those with significant complications of the liver cysts should be prioritized. Patients without renal insufficiency may receive a MELD score of 15 and those with renal insufficiency may receive a MELD score of 20. Additionally, patients may get 3 points every 3 months after reapplication.

d. Portal Hypertension

It is not uncommon for patients with liver cirrhosis to have bleeding from portal hypertension. Usually those bleeding episodes are controlled endoscopically. Patients with refractory portal hypertensive gastrointestinal bleeding should be prioritized for liver transplantation, although no additional points are added to the MELD scores of these patients.

e. Hepatopulmonary Syndrome (see Chapter 6)

f. Portopulmonary Hypertension (see Chapter 6)

g. Acute Budd-Chiari syndrome

Patients who present with acute Budd-Chiari syndrome tend to present similarly to acute/fulminant liver failure. Those patients are usually listed as Status 1A—meaning high priority for liver transplantation.

h. Primary Hyperoxaluria

Patients with primary hyperoxaluria who qualify for the MELD score exception must have liver biopsy proven alanine glycoxylate aminotransferase deficiency and must not have significant renal injury. In cases of significant renal injury, patients can only get the exception MELD score if they are listed for a combined liver-kidney transplant.

i. Familial Amyloidotic Polyneuropathy

Patients with familial amyloidotic polyneuropathy who are ambulatory and who have a modified body mass index greater than 700 are eligible candidates for the MELD score exception. For patients with extensive cardiac involvement with amyloid, patients should either be considered for a combined heart-liver transplant or neither.

j. Cystic Fibrosis

Cystic fibrosis tends to affect the liver, as apparent in Figure 12.2, which shows a nodular cirrhotic liver with widened fissures. No additional MELD score points are given for cystic fibrosis patients who have well-compensated lung disease. Patients with decompensated pulmonary function

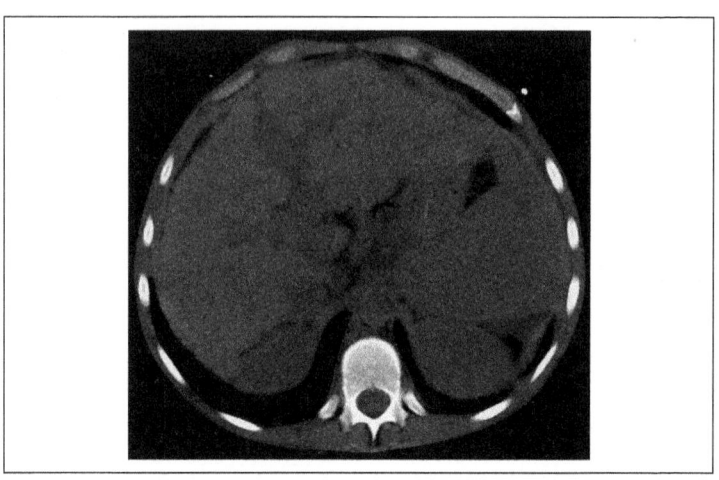

Figure 12.2. Cystic fibrosis leading to liver cirrhosis as evidenced by the nodular liver and widened fissures.

and who are listed for a combined lung and liver transplant qualify for an upgrade in their MELD score to 40.

k. Cholangiocarcinoma

Some patients with cholangiocarcinoma qualify for the MELD exception score. For patients to get the points, a protocol must be submitted to UNOS from the transplant center requesting the exception. The protocol is strict and addresses the specific pathology, prior neo-adjuvant therapy, surgical candidacy for partial hepatectomy, and the presence of lymphade-nopathy or regional metastatic disease, among other factors.

l. Primary Sclerosing Cholangitis

There are criteria that allow certain patients with recurrent bacterial cho-langitis to qualify for a MELD upgrade. The most common cause of bil-iary structural disease leading to recurrent bacterial cholangitis is PSC (Fig. 12.3). Patients who have two culture-proven bacteremias within a 6-month period or those patients who have septic complications of bacterial cholan-gitis qualify for the MELD upgrade. No special considerations are given to those patients with pruritis alone.

m. Hepatocellular Carcinoma

One of the approved exceptions pertains to the presence of hepatocellular carcinoma (HCC). More than 20,000 individuals were diagnosed with HCC in 2009. Although patients with HCC may have a low MELD indicating a low short-term mortality, the risk of waiting on the transplant list till their MELD increases will be at the expense of tumor progression, possibly to an extent where they no longer are candidates for transplantation because of metastatic disease. For this reason, UNOS has now broadened their

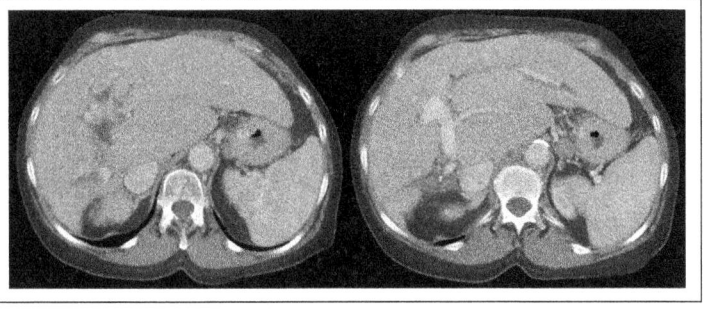

Figure 12.3. Liver cirrhosis from PSC as evidenced by biliary ductal dilation and the beads-on-a-string pattern.

recommendations pertaining to HCC in that a candidate with an HCC tumor that is 2 cm or greater and 5 cm or less or no more than 3 lesions, the largest being less than 3 cm in size (Stage T2 tumors), may be registered at a MELD score equivalent to a 15% probability of candidate death within 3 months. Currently, the patient is assigned a MELD score of 22 with an additional 3 points every 3 months on the wait list.

n. Miscellaneous Situations

At this time, the unusual liver tumors that may qualify for additional priority listing include hepatic epithelioid hemangioendotheliomas and hepatic adenomas in the presence of glycogen storage disease.

Patients who develop graft versus host disease after a living donor transplantation from small-for-size syndrome receive priority listing if they meet four of the six criteria pertaining to their laboratory values (serum bilirubin ≥10mg/dL, INR ≥1.5) or the presence of bile duct ischemia/leak, ascites, abnormal liver biopsy (centrilobular ballooning, necrosis, and cholestasis), or if the patient's symptoms started to develop at 5 days of the transplantation or after.

It is important to keep in mind the uncommon metabolic liver diseases that may qualify for MELD score upgrades. Those cases have to be individualized.

Hereditary hemorrhagic telengectasia or Rendu-Osler-Weber syndrome patients do not qualify for automatic MELD score upgrades. Those patients who develop acute biliary necrosis should be eligible for a MELD score of 40, whereas those who develop intractable heart failure should be eligible for a MELD score of 22.

The right time for referral for liver transplant evaluation is very critical and key in managing those ill patients. In patients with chronic liver disease and subsequent cirrhosis, evaluation should ensue once patients manifest at least one of the signs of liver decompensation, such as ascites, gastrointestinal bleeding from portal hypertension, Hepatorenal syndrome, portosystemic encephalopathy, or the development of hepatocellular carcinoma. The American Association for the Study of Liver Disease (AASLD) recommends that referral for liver transplantation should occur in patients with a MELD score equal to 10 or greater and a Child's Class B or more, or at the time of a patient's first major complication.

In acute/fulminant liver failure, referral for liver transplantation should occur as soon as the patient is admitted to the hospital. It is important to realize that patients with liver disease have a narrow window during which they are acceptable liver recipient candidates. Those patients are very tenuous, and waiting too long for transplantation results in the loss of their only opportunity for survival. Table 12.3 displays the most common indications for liver transplantation, and Figure 12.4 shows the proportion of each indication from 1992 to 2007.

Chronic Liver Disease

Alcohol-Related Liver Disease

The most common etiology of liver cirrhosis in Western countries is alcohol-related liver disease. It accounts for almost 12% of liver transplantations. The

Table 12.3 Indications of Liver Transplantation
Chronic liver disease
- Alcohol-related liver disease
- Hepatitis C-induced liver disease
- Hepatitis B-induced liver disease
- Nonalcoholic fatty liver disease
- Cholestatic liver disease
-> Primary biliary cirrhosis
-> Primary sclerosing cholangitis
- Other causes
-> Metabolic such as Wilson's disease, hemochromatosis, and primary hyperoxaluria
-> Autoimmune such as autoimmune hepatitis
-> Vascular such as Budd-Chiari, sinusoidal obstruction syndrome, and hypercoagulable states
-> Miscellaneous including adult polycystic liver disease, cystic fibrosis, and post-BMT graft vs. host disease
Acute/fulminant liver failure
- Acetaminophen-induced
- Acute viral hepatitis
- Drug-induced such as alcohol, halothane, isoniazid, phenytoin, rifampin, NSAIDs, amiodarone, sulfonamide, etc.
- Vascular causes such as portal vein thrombosis, Budd-Chiari, ischemic hepatitis, and veno-occlusive disease
- Metabolic such as acute fatty liver of pregnancy and Wilson's disease
Malignancy
- Hepatocellular carcinoma
- Cholangiocarcinoma

NSAIDs: nonsteroidal anti-inflammatory drugs; BMT: bone marrow transplant

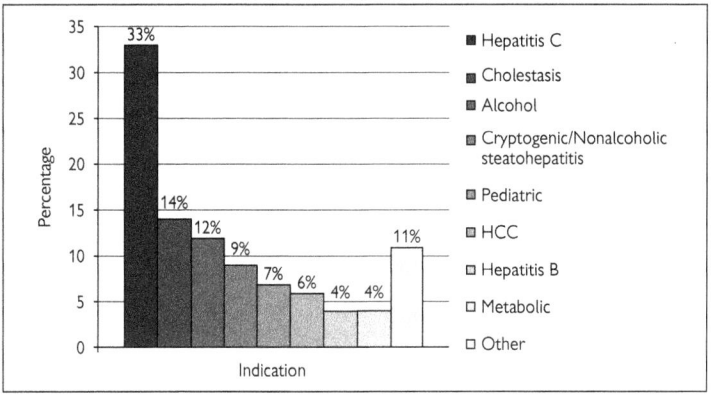

Figure 12.4. Proportion of indications for liver transplantation between 1992 and 2007. HCC: hepatocellular carcinoma

presence of alcoholic liver disease usually occurs in conjunction with chronic hepatitis C-induced liver disease, and it actually accounts for rapid progression to cirrhosis in those patients. Prior to listing for transplantation, patients with alcoholic cirrhosis must be abstinent from alcohol for at least 6 months, although many transplant centers push for longer duration of abstinence. The patients must have insight about their disease and must be aware and understand that their illness results from their alcoholism. They must be involved in a formal rehabilitation program with the involvement of either a psychiatrist or a psychologist to treat any underlying psychiatric illnesses. In addition, those patients must have a strong social support system. Although those patients are closely monitored and counseled prior to liver transplantation, 20% to 40% of them resume drinking alcohol after transplantation. Interestingly, the outcomes of patients with alcoholic liver cirrhosis post-transplantation are great with excellent graft and patients survival rates, which are higher for the patients who do not relapse into alcoholism.

Hepatitis C-Induced Liver Disease

Although alcoholic liver disease is the most common cause of liver disease, hepatitis C-induced liver cirrhosis is the most common indication for liver transplantation, accounting for almost one-third of all liver transplantations. Almost 5 million persons are infected with hepatitis C in the United States, of whom 4 million are chronic infections. Approximately 1 million of those patients will ultimately develop liver cirrhosis. Patients with hepatitis C-induced liver cirrhosis are at a higher risk for the development of HCC compared to the other causes of chronic liver disease. Unlike patients who are transplanted for alcohol-related liver disease, the outcomes of patients who are transplanted for hepatitis C-induced liver cirrhosis are not as promising, the reason being the risk of graft re-infection with hepatitis C. Reports have demonstrated that nearly all patients who have detectable viral levels will re-infect the graft. This is why attempts should be made to treat all hepatitis C-infected patients, preferably prior to the onset of fibrosis. Unlike patients with liver transplantation for hepatitis B cirrhosis, there are no empiric prophylactic therapies that patients can receive after transplantation. The burden of recurrent hepatitis C infection in the transplanted graft remains. In such cases, most transplant centers opt to treat the recurrent hepatitis C infection in the graft when it is histologically significant as defined by grade 3 or 4 inflammation or at least stage 2 fibrosis. Many studies have linked a set of predictive factors to severe hepatitis C recurrence in the graft. Those factors include a hepatitis C genotype 1b, an elevated viral load before transplantation and up to 2 weeks after transplantation, older donor, non-White recipient, and recurrent episodes of acute cellular rejection, among many other factors. It is important that the patient is aware of the possible risk of recurrence in the graft and the possibility of fibrosing cholestatic hepatitis, which holds an extremely high mortality at 1 year. The current antiviral agents used for the management of recurrent hepatitis C are a combination of alpha-interferon and ribavirin. With the availability of newer protease inhibitors (i.e., telaprevir and boceprevir), the management of recurrent hepatitis C post-liver transplantation would be greatly enhanced once they are approved for this indication.

Hepatitis B-Induced Liver Disease

The incidence of hepatitis B-induced cirrhosis is declining because of the adequate antiviral therapy available for treating those infections. For those patients who require transplantation, a major concern in transplanting patients with hepatitis B pertains to graft re-infection with recurrent hepatitis B. Predictors of re-infection include the patient's infectivity status in the pre-transplant state as measured by the patient's hepatitis B e antigen and the hepatitis B DNA level. Chronic hepatitis B patients require long-term prophylactic antiviral therapy post-transplantation to minimize the risk of graft re-infection with hepatitis B. Efforts continue to be directed at finding the best regimen to prevent re-infection. Currently, indefinite therapy with high-dose hepatitis B immunoglobulin in addition to lamivudine, a nucleoside analog, have been shown to decrease the rate of graft re-infection; however, with the availability of newer nucleoside/nucleotide agents such as entecavir and tenofovir, the duration of use of hepatitis B immunoglobulin could be potentially shortened.

Nonalcoholic Fatty Liver Disease

Nonalcoholic fatty liver disease, previously referred to as cryptogenic liver disease, remains to be a major cause of liver cirrhosis and an indication for liver transplantation. Patients with nonalcoholic fatty liver disease tend to be obese, hyperlipidemic, and suffer from diabetes mellitus or insulin resistance. Targeted efforts at weight loss and control of the comorbidities including hyperlipidemia and diabetes mellitus remain to be key at managing such patients before and after liver transplantation. Graft failure is uncommon despite the likelihood of nonalcoholic steatohepatitis recurrence in the graft.

Cholestatic Liver Diseases—Primary Biliary Cirrhosis and Primary Sclerosing Cholangitis

Both primary biliary cirrhosis (PBC) and primary sclerosing cholangitis (PSC) are diseases of the biliary tree that result in cholestasis and subsequent liver failure. Their only cure is liver transplantation. The outcomes post-transplantation are successful, but there always is a risk that the disease will recur in the transplanted graft—more so in the PSC patients, with recurrence rates reaching 20%. Generally PBC patients start to decline as they develop hyperbilirubinemia. Patients with PSC tend to develop recurrent bouts of biliary sepsis caused by biliary obstruction. Those patients may become dependent on biliary drains. At certain transplant centers, patients with PSC qualify for the MELD upgrade. Patients with PSC tend to be not adequately served by the MELD scoring system. Given the risk of development of cholangiocarcinoma in this patient population, consideration should be given to the use of living donor liver transplantation.

Other Liver Diseases

Any long-standing metabolic, genetic, auto-immune, or even vascular disease that impacts the liver may result in ESLD and, therefore, the need for a liver transplantation. Metabolic disorders such as hemochromatosis and Wilson's disease may result in liver cirrhosis, and their only cure is liver transplantation. The neurological complications associated with Wilson's disease are reversible after liver transplantation. Urgent liver transplantation is indicated for patients who present with a Wilsonian crisis. Although patients with primary hyperoxaluria develop renal end-organ damage, rather than liver damage, the defect is hepatic, so those patients require a combined kidney-liver transplantation. The first-line treatment for patients with auto-immune hepatitis includes steroids and immunomodulators. In certain instances, failure to medically control the inflammation leads to liver cirrhosis and the need for liver transplantation. Despite the excellent outcome, those patients are at a higher risk of acute cellular rejection post transplantation. Patients with Budd-Chiari syndrome have obstruction of their hepatic vein, leading to liver congestion and a presentation very similar to decompensated chronic liver disease with ascites and portal hypertension. The decision to transplant those patients versus performing a transjugular intrahepatic porto-systemic shunt or a surgical shunt depends on the liver biopsy histology. Other indications for liver transplantation include adult polycystic disease, glycogen storage diseases, amyloidosis, and sarcoidosis.

Acute Liver Failure or Fulminant Hepatic Failure

Early recognition is critical for appropriate management of patients with acute liver failure. Acute liver failure is defined as sudden severe liver injury in a patient with a normal liver (with the exception of patients with Wilson's disease or chronic hepatitis B infection). Those patients have an impaired hepatic synthetic function and manifest with hepatic encephalopathy over the course of 8 weeks or less. Patients with underlying chronic liver disease may decompensate and tend to present similarly to patients with acute liver failure. This condition is referred to as acute chronic liver failure (ACLF). Although some acute liver failure patients tend to survive and spontaneously recover, many others require liver transplantation. The King's College Criteria help decide which patients will need a liver transplantation as demonstrated in Figure 12.5. Acetaminophen toxicity accounts for the majority of acute liver failure cases (40%), of whom 65% spontaneously recover. Complications of ACLF include hepatic encephalopathy, ranging from mild confusion and slurred speech (grade I) as well as moderate confusion and lethargy (grade II), to marked confusion, incoherence, and obtunded state (grade III), to the comatose state (grade IV). Other complications include the more serious cerebral edema, which occurs in up to 80% of patients with grade IV hepatic encephalopathy; acute renal failure, which is encountered in up to 50% of patients with acute liver failure; metabolic disturbances; infections; and sepsis. In those patients who require a liver transplant, emergent liver transplantation leads to excellent outcomes with 1-year survival rates higher than 80%, especially when performed before the detrimental irreversible neurological complications from cerebral edema are encountered. For this reason, patients presenting with ACLF should be automatically transferred to specialized liver transplantation centers for adequate intracranial pressure monitoring and appropriate intensive care management.

Liver Malignancy—Hepatocellular Carcinoma and Cholangiocarcinoma

Hepatocellular carcinoma accounts for up to 90% of all liver malignancies. The incidence of HCC has been on the rise over the past few decades mainly because of the increasing rates of chronic hepatitis C infections and also because of obesity, diabetes mellitus, and liver cirrhosis. In the MELD era, HCC continues to be a rising indication for liver transplantation. Although liver transplantation offers definitive treatment for patients with HCC, very careful patient selection must be implemented prior to referring patients for liver transplantation. Prelisting

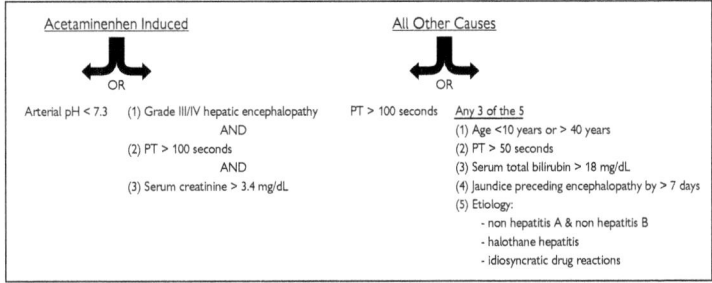

Figure 12.5. Liver transplantation for acute liver failure—King's College Criteria.

PT: prothrombin time

work up focuses on excluding the presence of metastatic disease and vascular invasion by obtaining computed tomography (CT) scans of the chest, abdomen, and pelvis in addition to a bone scan. Patients who meet the Milan criteria are considered candidates for liver transplantation. Based on prior studies, the 5-year patient and graft survival for patients is comparable to patients without HCC. The criteria take the number of lesions and the size of the lesions into account and assumes that there is no vascular invasion, no metastatic disease, and no tumor infiltration. A solitary tumor less than 5 cm in largest diameter or a total of three tumors with none being larger than 3 cm in size is still considered within Milan criteria. Patients who meet Milan criteria receive extra points toward their MELD score to increase their priority on the liver transplantation list, as detailed above in the MELD exception section. This upgrade results from the concern that waiting for protracted time periods on the transplantation list may result in metastasis and increased tumor burden. For patients who were just slightly outside Milan criteria, aggressive directed therapy in attempts to shrink the tumor (i.e., downstaging) such as radiofrequency ablation, chemoembolization, and radiation therapy followed by listing remains controversial. There is a regional variation with respect to the use of Milan criteria, with certain regions using extended criteria such as the University of California San Francisco (UCSF) criteria: single tumor 6.5 cm or smaller, maximum of three total tumors with none greater than 4.5 cm, and cumulative tumor size 8 cm or smaller.

To date, the best management of cholangiocarcinoma remains to be determined. Studies have shown that the outcomes of transplanted patients have been very poor, with very high recurrence of cholangiocarcinoma. Recently, however, patients with hilar cholangiocarcinoma have demonstrated acceptable 5-year survival rates, especially when receiving multimodal therapy with chemotherapy and radiation therapy. Therefore, hilar cholangiocarcinoma is observed to be a relative contraindication for transplantation, whereas other cholangiocarcinomas are absolute contraindications.

Contraindications for Liver Transplantation

Contraindications for liver transplantation may be absolute or relative, as demonstrated in Table 12.4. Absolute contraindications imply that the patients have certain conditions that would complicate the course of their liver transplantation, making the likelihood of a successful outcome very slim.

Relative contraindications, on the other hand, are more lenient, as they include certain suboptimal conditions that decrease the chance of a successful outcome. Different transplant centers have their own relative contraindications depending on the number of liver transplantation cases performed, the transplant surgeon's level of expertise, as well as the presence of ongoing clinical trials at the centers. Relative contraindications tend to change over time depending on the advancements made to deal with certain comorbid illnesses such as co-infection with human immunodeficiency virus, as well as new surgical techniques that

Table 12.4 Contraindications of Liver Transplantation

Absolute
- Active extrahepatic malignancy
- Hepatocellular carcinoma outside Milan criteria
- Angiosarcoma
- Active substance abuse (alcohol, narcotic use, recreational drug use)
- Severe cardiopulmonary disease
- Active and uncontrolled infections and sepsis
- Anatomic barriers leading to surgical technical challenge
- Morbid Obesity (BMI >40 kg/m^2)
- Noncompliance
Relative
- Prior extrahepatic malignancy—now cured
- Age
- Portal vein thrombosis
- Cholangiocarcinoma
- Human immunodeficiency viral infection
- Chronic or refractory infections
- Poor social support
- Active psychiatric illnesses

BMI: body mass index

develop to deal with variants in anatomy and complications such as portal vein thrombosis. Despite the variations in the relative contraindications between different centers, all centers seem to be in consensus with regards to the absolute contraindications for liver transplantation.

Absolute Contraindications

Active extrahepatic malignancy is an absolute contraindication to liver transplantation. Those patients with HCC are considered for liver transplantation if they are within the Milan criteria. Angiosarcoma of the liver is very aggressive and remains to be an absolute contraindication for liver transplantation. Active substance abuse, be it alcohol, recreational drugs, or narcotics, is an absolute contraindication to liver transplantation. At most centers, patients must be "drug-free" for at least 6 months prior to liver transplantation. Patients with a history of substance abuse are usually referred to a psychiatrist to help them cope with their addiction and are also advised to join detoxification programs. It is not unusual for patients to have random drug screen testing during their clinic visits. Cigarette smoking is not a contraindication, but it is strongly advised against, as it not only increases the risk of malignancy in general, but it also increases the risk of hepatic artery thrombosis. Severe cardiopulmonary disease is an absolute contraindication for liver transplantation, as those patients have a high intra-operative and post-operative mortality. Those patients do not tolerate the operation, and if they survive the surgery, they tend to have a protracted and prolonged post-surgical course with many post-operative complications, including worsening heart failure and mechanical ventilation dependence. Targeted tests including transthoracic echocardiograms and dobutamine stress tests, and at times right heart catheterizations, are performed in the pre-operative testing to identify those patients with Hepatopulmonary syndrome and those with portopulmonary hypertension. Active and uncontrolled infections are an absolute contraindication to transplantation and must be adequately treated prior to subjecting patients to major surgery followed by immunosuppression therapy. Some anatomical barriers may exist, precluding the ability of the surgeons to perform a liver transplantation. Such cases include extensive thrombosis of the entire portal and superior mesenteric venous systems. At specialized centers, few surgeons tend to perform extensive vascular reconstruction to facilitate patient listing for liver transplantation. Morbid obesity defined as a body mass index greater than 40 kg/m^2 is considered a contraindication for liver transplantation, as it carries a high post-operative mortality rates. Certain psychosocial factors such as noncompliance are considered absolute contraindications for liver transplantation, as failure to comply with medications post-transplantation will almost definitely lead to rejection and a wasted precious organ.

Relative Contraindications

As mentioned above, active extrahepatic malignancy is an absolute contraindication to liver transplantation. On the contrary, prior history of malignancy that has been treated and is now cured is a relative contraindication. Listing depends on the type of tumor, stage at diagnosis, prior therapy or surgery, and the duration of "cancer-free" state. It is preferable for those patients to be evaluated by an oncologist prior to listing. Most patients have to be "cancer-free" for at least 2 years prior to listing, but longer periods are preferred for patients with history of colon cancer, breast cancer, and malignant melanoma. Generally, if it is determined that a patient's risk of cancer recurrence is less than 10% in 5 years, transplantation is acceptable. Age is a relative contraindication for liver transplantation. It is without a doubt that younger patients tend to tolerate major operations better than elderly patients; however, assessment of physiological fitness would be more appropriate in patient selection. The presence of a portal vein thrombosis is considered a relative contraindication for transplantation. Its presence definitely poses a challenge complicating the technicality of the surgery; however, depending on the expertise of the transplant surgeons and the extent of the thrombosis, the surgery can still be performed. Cholangiocarcinoma remains to be a relative contraindication for liver transplantation given the poor outcome resulting from high recurrence rates. Human immunodeficiency viral infections place patients at a higher risk for complications; however, with adequate therapy with highly active antiretroviral therapy, the post-transplantation outcomes of HIV patients is similar to those without HIV. Patients with HIV will require closer monitoring in the post-transplant period because many immunosuppressive drugs have been found to interact with the antiretroviral drugs. Some patients harbor chronic infections that are refractory to standard therapy, including osteomyelitis and pulmonary fungal infections. Those patients are a relative contraindication for transplantation. Each of those cases should be personalized prior to making a decision about listing. Having an optimal social support structure for patients undergoing liver transplantation is an important component in the outcome of liver transplantation. Similarly, certain psychiatric illnesses that can be resolved over time and with expert intervention are not absolute but, rather, relative contraindications for liver transplantation.

Selected References

Cho SM, Murugan R, & Al-Khafaji A. Fulminant Hepatic Failure In Fink MP, Abraham E, Vincent JL, and Kochanek P, ed. *Textbook of Critical Care*, Saunders, 6th Edition 2010.

O'Leary JG, Lepe R, & Davis GL. Indications for liver transplantation.*Gastroenterology*. 2008;134(6):1764–1776. Review.

Starzl TE, Shunzaburo I, Van Thiel DH, et al. Evolution of Liver Transplantation. *Hepatology* 1982;2(5):614–636.

Chapter 13

An Approach to Anesthesia for Liver Transplantation

Charles Boucek

Liver transplantation has evolved from an experimental procedure to a life-saving therapeutic option for patients with end-stage liver disease (ESLD). The procedure remains challenging from both a surgical and anesthetic viewpoint, requiring a major commitment of resources. Candidates for liver transplantation ordinarily undergo extensive pre-operative testing to assure that they have irremediable liver failure, that all other medical conditions are optimized, and that conditions that preclude successful outcome are absent.

Timing of liver transplantation is determined by the availability of graft organs. Liver transplantation may occur at any time of day and is frequently started at night. Organ donation may occur in a hospital remote from the transplantation center. To prevent disruption of planned operations, organs are often harvested at the end of the elective surgical schedule. Transportation of organs to the transplant center, serological testing for transmissible diseases, examination of the graft, and back-table preparation all contribute to cold ischemia time. Despite use of preservation solutions and reduced temperature (ice bath), organ function deteriorates as ischemia time increases. Therefore, liver transplantation (other than from living related donors) is an emergency operation. Recipients should be fully evaluated pre-operatively to prevent unnecessary delays once a suitable organ is available.

Pre-operative evaluation of candidates for liver transplantation occurs at two occasions: initially when evaluating the candidate for inclusion on the transplant list ("listing") and again immediately pre-operatively when interventions and additional testing are limited by time constraints. During the screening evaluation, patients are referred to the transplantation center by their primary physician, gastroenterologist, or hepatologist. They are evaluated by a surgeon and other specialists as needed including a social worker, psychiatrist, anesthesiologist and other consultants as indicated. Workup generally includes a history and physical, laboratory testing for biochemical function and determination of the model for end-stage liver disease (MELD), imaging of liver volume, and assessment for malignancy. Pulmonary function tests, imaging studies (chest X-ray, abdominal CT), and arterial blood gasses (as indicated) are reviewed. Careful evaluation of cardiovascular function is especially important. In addition to an

EKG, a stress echocardiogram or similar test is usually warranted because ESLD may result in pathological vasodilation requiring extremely high cardiac output, especially during reperfusion of the graft. Limited cardiac reserve resulting from right heart failure, ischemic disease, valvular stenosis, unstable rhythm, or pulmonary hypertension may lead to cardiovascular collapse during the stress of reperfusion. If a stress echocardiogram is equivocal, then a nuclear cardiology study (adenosine-thallium scan) or heart catheterization may be performed.

Immediate Pre-Operative Evaluation

Candidates for liver transplantation are admitted to the hospital when a potentially suitable graft organ becomes available. In the immediate pre-operative period, it is important to obtain consent for the procedure and confirm availability of blood products.

Liver transplantation has three stages, each with distinct physiology and clinical challenges.

Stage one: The pre-anhepatic stage starts with induction of anesthesia through removal of the native liver.

Stage two: The anhepatic stage is the period from removal of the native liver to reperfusion of the graft.

Stage three: The neo-hepatic stage starts with reperfusion through the end of surgery.

Stage one events include induction of anesthesia, establishment of vascular access and monitors, provision for venous return during manipulation of the inferior vena cava, and devascularization of the liver and hepatectomy. Physiological changes of ELSD include vasodilation, increased cardiac output, and increased SvO2. End-stage liver disease often manifests focal areas of vasodilation unresponsive to catecholamines. Administration of vasoconstrictors may transiently increase blood pressure but often leads to steal physiology; vasoplegic areas remain vasodilated and vascularly responsive tissue becomes ischemic.

Stage one issues include maintenance of appropriate intravascular volume, treatment of progressive metabolic acidosis, and hypocalcemia. Hypotension during this period can result from drainage of ascites, bleeding, hypocalcemia, and obstruction of venous return. Correction of intravascular volume and ionized calcium levels should occur before adding a vasopressor or ionotrope. Hypotension unresponsive to volume and calcium or the occurrence of significant fibrinolysis (by thromboelastogram) is unusual during this stage and may indicate an unrecognized bacteremia.

Induction of Anesthesia

At least one absolutely reliable IV should be established; for frail or unstable patients, a radial arterial line may be placed using local anesthesia prior to induction. Liver transplantation patients should be considered to have a full stomach if they have ascites even if they have not recently eaten and will usually require rapid-sequence induction. Awake intubation, fiberoptic or otherwise, may be needed for patients with a difficult airway, recognizing that the coagulopathies common in liver failure may complicate even mildly traumatic intubation attempts. Induction medications may include etomidate, narcotics, benzodiazepines, thiopental, or propofol with appropriate dosing; succinylcholine, rocuronium, or other non-depolarizing muscle relaxants can be used, recognizing that agents requiring hepatic metabolism will have a prolonged effect. Ventilation with air/oxygen and a sub-MAC concentration of an inhalation agent is usually well tolerated. Nitrous oxide should be avoided. Isoflurane, sevoflurane, and desflurane have all been used successfully; halothane should probably be avoided because of potential toxicity for the graft. An adequate mechanical ventilator is essential because liver transplantation is a long procedure and multiple factors may compromise pulmonary function, including ascites, pleural effusions, ventilation perfusion mismatching, and pulmonary vascular abnormalities.

Routine monitors of temperature, neuromuscular function, capnography, pulse oximetry, ventilation gasses, and blood pressure should be used during induction. After both arterial lines are placed, the blood pressure cuff and all bracelets should be removed to prevent limb ischemia from tourniquet effect should limb swelling occur. Urinary and gastric drainage catheters should be inserted with care. Nasal bleeding can be brisk and require packing. The gastric drainage catheter should remain in place along with the transesophageal echocardiography (TEE), if one is used. Despite the frequent presence of esophageal varices, TEE provides valuable information. The probe should be inserted with care and generous quantities of lubricant. Transesophageal echocardiography should probably be avoided in patients who have recently (within the last 2 weeks) had banding of varices or have a history of other esophageal pathology.

Placement of the vascular catheters needed for liver transplantation using local anesthesia is more than most patients can tolerate while awake. Standard vascular access includes two arterial lines so that continuous blood pressure monitoring is not interrupted during sampling of arterial blood. Simultaneous attempts at line placement by multiple individuals may increase the risk of inadvertent needle stick injury; it is important that one provider vigilantly observe the patient and vital signs during the placement of invasive monitors. A femoral arterial line, if placed, should be below the inguinal ligament. Femoral and radial arterial pressures may be similar during the early phases of liver transplantation, but following reperfusion, femoral arterial lines provide more reliable pressure measurement. Standard venous access in our institution includes placement of a veno-venous bypass cannula if bypass is being considered, an introducer to accommodate a PA catheter, an infusion line for vasoactive medications and two dedicated volume lines, each capable of supporting blood infusions at 400 mL/min. A dedicated line for infusion of buffer (sodium bicarbonate or tromethamine [THAM]) is useful to treat the progressive metabolic acidosis that accompanies hepatectomy. The veno-venous bypass cannula may be placed percutaneously in the right internal jugular vein. Large bore venous lines may be placed in the right and left internal jugular, external jugular, and antecubital veins. Frequently the right internal jugular vein can accommodate both a bypass cannula and the introducer for the PA catheter. It is recommended that these be placed through separate insertion sites approximately 1 to 2 cm apart, with both bare wires inserted before either the cannula or introducer is placed to reduce the risk of shearing or puncturing an existing plastic catheter with the second needle. A right ventricular ejection pulmonary artery catheter (REF) that has the capacity to measure CVP and PA pressures, SvO2, continuous thermodilution cardiac output, right ventricular end diastolic volume, and right ventricular ejection fraction is especially useful.

Venous Return

Simple cross-clamping of the suprahepatic inferior vena cava usually is not tolerated in adults. The hepatic vein(s) may be controlled by careful dissection and a side clamp that permits continued flow through the retro-hepatic vena cava. There is always some sequestration of volume below the clamp, increasing fluid/transfusion requirements and resulting in hypervolemia when the clamps are removed in Stage three. Additionally, return of blood from the splanchnic circulation may require a temporary portosystemic shunt. Another approach is to establish a veno–venous bypass circuit. A drainage cannula is advanced into the iliac vein and another placed into the portal vein; these are joined by a Y connection. Blood is returned to a cannula placed in the jugular or axillary vein using an in-line pump. The circuit does not include a reservoir, oxygenator, heat exchanger, or bubble detector. The circuit is heparin bonded, and full systemic heparinization is not necessary, although small doses of heparin (two to three thousand units IV) can be given for patients at higher risk of thromboembolism (primary biliary cirrhosis, hepatocelluar carcinoma, or hypercoagulable thrombelastography [TEG]). Flow rate through the circuit is monitored; rates below 2 L/min increase the risk of clot formation. If flow through the circuit is inadequate, then repositioning of the drainage cannulas and increasing intravascular volume may improve flow. When bypass is initiated, the anesthesia providers should look for sudden changes in vital signs, facial swelling, and Bispectral index (BIS), if available, and should view the right atrium and ventricle by TEE. Turbulent flow in the right heart should resolve within seconds; persistent echogenic turbulence should raise the suspicion of air entrainment into the circuit. Bypass may be continued into Stage three using the iliac drainage. Portal blood flow will be removed from the circuit and directed into the graft organ prior to reperfusion. Maintaining veno-venous bypass into Stage three restores cardiac preload, reduces venous engorgement of the surgical field, and permits temporary reapplication of clamps if there is major post-reperfusion bleeding from the retro-hepatic cava. A variant circuit using the portal vein without iliac cannulation usually has lower flow rates and requires termination of bypass prior to graft reperfusion.

Maintenance of Anesthesia

Maintenance of anesthesia is usually accomplished using a sub-MAC concentration of an inhalation agent supplemented by narcotics with the addition of a benzodiazepine to assure amnesia. A BIS monitor can be useful to assess depth of anesthesia. Continuous manipulation of the concentration of the inhalation agent based on blood pressure is not appropriate because transient hypotension usually does not result from anesthetic overdose but, rather, from events in the surgical field. Discontinuation of the inhalation agent is unlikely to resolve the hypotension and raises the prospect of intra-operative recall. Discontinuation of inhalation agents and reliance on total intravenous anesthesia (TIVA) techniques may be utilized when indicated. Generous doses of narcotics, benzodiazepines, and muscle relaxants may be given despite the presumed reduction of hepatic clearance. Clearance of anesthetic agents is a concern if extubation at the end of surgery is planned. This may apply to carefully selected patients with minimal comorbidities, ideal donor organs, and uneventful surgery. For most patients, post-operative mechanical ventilation is expected; although the native liver may have poor drug clearance, the graft organ will function better. If it does not (primary graft non-function), then continued ICU monitoring and mechanical ventilation will be needed regardless of medications administered.

Assessment of Volume

Throughout the operation, immediate correction of intravascular volume is critical for success. Bleeding, massive loss of third space fluid, and sequestration of circulating volume all can result in hypovolemia. Overly vigorous volume replacement or the sudden increase in venous return that accompanies restoration of the infra-and supra- hepatic *vena cava* during reperfusion, can result in volume overload with increased bleeding, hepatic congestion, stress on venous anastomoses, and greater difficulty with graft manipulation. Correction of hypovolemia after it occurs is not adequate. Proactive prevention of stressful episodes (hypotension) is critical. Although initial episodes of hypotension may respond to resuscitative measures, subsequent episodes are not tolerated as well, with increasing multisystem dysfunction. A combination of CVP, PA diastolic pressure, SvO2, right vertricular end diastolic volume[1], pulse pressure variation (PPV), stroke volume variation (SVV), observation of the filling of the heart by TEE, and observation of the surgical field are all useful to assess intravascular volume. Neither measured hematocrit nor estimated blood loss are reliable guides; the former is affected by ascites formation, whereas the latter is limited by error of measurement (+/-10%) that frequently exceeds total circulating volume. Urine output is reassuring when it is present, but administration of diuretics makes this an unreliable monitor of volume. Many transplantation patients require renal replacement therapy. Adequate vascular access, available blood products, and a suitable infusion device are needed to replace circulating volume at the rate that it is being lost.

Progressive metabolic acidosis occurs as the native liver is devascularized. Treatment with sodium bicarbonate, although effective, may be limited by the ability to increase ventilation or by rising serum sodium levels. To reduce the risk of central pontine myelinolysis, serum sodium levels should not change more than 10 meq over 24 hours. Tromethamine is an alternative buffer that contains no sodium and, therefore, will reduce sodium levels. Both THAM and sodium bicarbonate may be used in combination to maintain stable pH and sodium levels. If THAM is not available, then an infusion of 5% dextrose with 3 ampoules of sodium bicarbonate added per liter may be infused to correct metabolic acidosis without increasing sodium levels; this may require large fluid volumes with the need for diuresis.

The second stage of liver transplantation starts with removal of the native liver. There is a slight decrease in cardiac demand when the liver is removed from circulation. During Stage two, citrate used as an anticoagulant in banked blood is not metabolized. The resulting citrate intoxication can result in reduced ionized calcium levels with hypotension and reduced cardiac contractility. Repeated infusions of calcium chloride are usually needed. For patients with hepatitis B, hepatitis B immune globulin (HBIG) may be infused after the native liver is removed and before placement of the graft in an effort to clear the virus. Pretreatment with antihistamine and/or corticosteroids is useful because HBIG infusion can cause hypotension—especially if given rapidly.

Preparation for Reperfusion

During Stage two, metabolic parameters should be corrected to optimal values. In anticipation of a potassium load at reperfusion, serum potassium should be maintained below 4 meq/L. Hyperventilation, forced diuresis, glucose/insulin infusions, washing of banked blood to remove potassium-rich residual plasma, and gastric suction may all be necessary to achieve this target. Serum glucose may fall when hepatic glycogen stores are not available. Serum glucose should be between 80 and 250 mg/dL. Hematocrit should be between 25% and 35 %. Lower values increase cardiac demand and reduce blood viscosity; high values may result in clotting of vessels. Base excess should be corrected as close to 0 as possible. Clotting function as manifested by TEG should be noted, but transfusion of blood products other than red cells and plasma and treatment with protamine or antifibrinolytics should be avoided to prevent thromboembolism. Hemodynamic manipulation during the end of Stage two may minimize problems at reperfusion. Methylene blue, a nitric oxide scavenger, has been shown to reduce catecholamine requirements and may improve shunting in hepatopulmonary syndrome. One mg/kg may be administered intravenously as a bolus. This will result in transient increase in blood pressure. Both SaO2 and SvO2 measurements will decrease as an artifact. In most patients, both values return to premethylene blue values within 5 minutes. Communication with the surgeon regarding the events of reperfusion is important. Many surgeons request immunosuppressant doses of corticosteroid prior to reperfusion, although the dose and timing varies. Patients who have positive lymphocytotoxic cross-match may have more difficult reperfusion and have a higher chance of early rejection. During Stage two, if veno-venous bypass is being used, the portal cannula will be discontinued to permit anastamosis of the portal vein to the graft. When the vascular anastamoses are nearly complete, the surgeon may "flush" the organ with the patient's blood by permitting inflow from the portal vein into the graft while the hepatic vein is still clamped. Blood flushes stagnant fluid from the graft onto the surgical field. In anticipation of reperfusion, systemic blood pressure should be increased so that a 30% decrease can be tolerated. Reperfusion may result in bradycardia when cold, anoxic, high-potassium fluid reaches the heart from the graft. Epinephrine, vasopressin, calcium, atropine, and equipment for defibrillation and/or cardiac pacing should be immediately available.

Stage three, the neo-hepatic stage, starts with reperfusion; blood flows from the portal circulation through the graft to the hepatic vein and the heart. Hypotension is common and can be multifactorial in etiology. The newly perfused organ becomes filled with blood, transiently unloading the mesenteric vasculature. Fluid returning from the graft to the heart is cold, has products of ischemic metabolism, and has residual preservation solution along with a variable quantity of clots and air bubbles. Reperfusion syndrome is a reduction in the systemic blood pressure of 30% or more occurring at this time. It is usually treated with epinephrine in rapidly escalating doses. Hypotension is often accompanied by bradycardia. If this results from acute hyperkalemia, then calcium is useful; otherwise epinephrine, atropine, external pacing, or cardiac massage may be used. Blood gasses and electrolytes should be obtained immediately after reperfusion (30 seconds) and at 5 minutes. Ionized calcium may be increased because of metabolism of citrate if the graft functions, unmasking the calcium load provided during Stage two. Rarely is hypercalcemia a persistent problem. Potassium level may be very high on the 30-second specimen but will rapidly correct if circulation can be maintained. Because venous return is more efficient, CVP may be acutely elevated from blood that had been sequestered below the clamps that have now been removed. Acute hypervolemia may require phlebotomy using syringes to aspirate blood from the venous lines. Blood removed may be placed in the cell saver or infusion pump reservoirs with suitable amounts of citrate to prevent clotting. Embolic or *in situ* development of intracardiac clots can occur during liver transplantation. Clots have been successfully treated with low-dose recombinant tissue plasminogen activator, but they may result in cardiac arrest.

If bleeding caused by injury to a blood vessel requires surgical hemostasis, administering platelets or activated clotting factors is a waste of resources and causes a risk of thrombotic and other complications. Bleeding from injury to the inferior vena cava can be massive and technically difficult to repair because of the location of the injury and the delicacy of the vessel wall. Retraction of the graft is often necessary to approach the bleeding site. Packing to tamponade bleeding can be used temporarily to permit volume replacement. Bleeding of 400 mL/min from a single site generally requires surgical intervention with replacement of blood volume to buy time. Diffuse bleeding without an identifiable site, may be due to a coagulopathy, hypothermia, and hypocalcemia that should be corrected.

Thrombelastography

A three-channel TEG is useful to direct administration of clot-stabilizing agents and blood products. Immediately post-reperfusion, a three-channel TEG should be obtained with a "natural" channel, a channel with added protamine, and a third channel with a anti-fibrinolytic agent such as epsilon amino caproic acid (AMICAR). The R-value is the time to first appearance of clotting. It represents the time required for platelet activation and is prolonged with heparin, deficiency of clotting factors and severe fibrinolysis. The alpha angle measures the rate of clot propagation and is responsive to platelet and cryoprecipitate administration. The maximum amplitude (MA) is a measure of clot strength and is most dependent on platelet number and function. The pattern of clot formation followed by MA decreasing to a flat line indicates fibrinolysis. Fibrinolysis may be diagnosed early if the AMICAR channel reacts more quickly and vigorously than the other channels. Documented fibrinolysis should be treated with small doses (250–500 mg IV) of AMICAR or other anti-fibrinolytics. Administering blood products without treating ongoing fibrinolysis wastes resources. Heparin effect may be seen from products released by the injured liver, even if no heparin has been administered. Protamine administration should be guided by the TEG. In some patients, especially when massive blood loss has been an ongoing problem, all three TEG channels will appear as flat lines. This indicates that clotting factors have been depleted. An often effective strategy is to treat with both AMICAR for fibrinolysis and protamine for heparin effect and then add platelets, cryoprecipitate, and fresh frozen plasma with further monitoring of TEG to guide therapy.

Small for Size Grafts

The normal liver has two blood supplies: portal venous blood and hepatic arterial blood. Liver grafts are usually reperfused with portal blood. A small for size graft may not be able to accommodate the flow from a dilated mesenteric circulation, resulting in graft engorgement. Reduction of portal flow may be accomplished pharmacologically with vasopressin, octreotide, or surgically by clamping the splenic artery.

Hepatic Artery

The hepatic artery is reconnected to supply oxygenated blood to the liver and biliary system. The biliary system depends on arterial blood. Untreated hepatic arterial thrombosis will result in biliary complication and eventual graft failure. A Doppler device may be used to assure continued arterial flow.

Biliary Reconstruction

Reconnection of the biliary system may be either duct-to-duct or may require a roux-en-y reconstruction depending on the anatomy involved. Roux-en-y reconstruction adds to the duration of surgery.

Assessment of Graft Function

Adequacy of graft function can be assessed in many ways. The graft color and the appearance are noteworthy. The production of bile is a strong positive indication of graft function. If the graft function is good, then blood gasses should trend toward normalization of pH, bicarbonate, lactate, osmolarity, and base excess. If glucose levels are high, then glucose levels should normalize with uptake to form glycogen and release of glucose from glycogen stores preventing hypoglycemia. Ionized calcium levels may temporarily increase because of metabolism of citrate. Twitch monitoring may indicate metabolism of muscle relaxants. If graft function is good, then maintenance of hemodyanamic stability should become easier. The need for escalating doses of catecholamines may indicate graft dysfunction unless some other problem has developed.

Abdominal Closure and ICU Transfer

Closure of the abdomen may be performed after adequate hemostasis. Rarely, intra-abdominal swelling requires delayed closure. Even with correct instrument counts, x ray films are useful to assure that needles and sponges have not been retained in the abdomen. The receiving ICU team should be informed of monitoring line, vasoactive agents, intra-operative events, and expected arrival time. Moving the patient to the ICU requires a team effort; portable monitoring, continuation of vasoactive agents, and sedation as well as manual ventilation are needed during transfer. Adequate monitoring and transfusion lines should be maintained in the immediate post-operative period in anticipation of possible need to return to the operating room.

High-Risk Patients

Certain conditions further complicate liver transplantation. These include fulminant hepatic failure, porto-pulmonary hypertension and portal vein thrombosis.

Fulminant hepatic failure most commonly result from acetaminophen overdose. The physiological compensations of ESLD may not be present, but intracranial hypertension from brain swelling is a major problem. This is often monitored invasively. Intubation with sedation and muscle relaxants, mechanical hyperventilation, elevation of the head, EEG burst suppression with barbituates, systemic cooling, hyperosmolar therapy with manitol, and hypertonic saline may be guided by measurement of intracranial pressure.

Patients with porto-pulmonary hypertension may develop right heart failure when increased cardiac output is needed.

Patients with portal vein thrombosis often have copius bleeding if thrombectomy is attempted. They may require multivisceral transplantation.

Selected References

Burtenshaw AJ & Isaac JL. The Role of Trans-Oesophogeal Echocardiography for Perioperative Cardiovascular Monitoring during Orthotopic Liver Transplantation. *Liver Transplantation* 2006;12:1577–1583.

Kang YG, Martin DJ, Marquez J, et al. Intraoperative Changes in Blood Coagulation and Thromboelastographic Monitoring in Liver Transplantationl *Anesth Analg.* 1985;64:888–896.

Chapter 14

Liver Transplant Surgical Techniques

Juan Mejia and Abhinav Humar

The surgical procedure of liver transplant has undergone numerous technical modifications and variations over the course of the last 30 years. It remains a technically demanding procedure with the potential for significant intra-operative complications. These relate to the magnitude of the procedure itself as well as the fact that it is usually performed in ill individuals with decompensated liver disease and the complications associated with that—most notably portal hypertension and coagulopathy. Nevertheless, with proper adherence to the basic steps, the procedure can be performed in the majority of these patients safely and effectively.

Adult Deceased Donor Liver Transplant

Hepatectomy

The surgical procedure begins with the removal of the recipient's native diseased liver, as in the vast majority of cases, liver transplant is performed in an orthotopic fashion. The abdominal cavity is entered via bilateral subcostal incisions with a midline extension, if needed. The hilar structures are dissected, starting with the hepatic artery, which is divided as high as possible. If the common hepatic artery is of small caliber at this level, then it can be traced proximally to the gastroduodenal artery or splenic artery at the time of anastomosis. The common bile duct is then identified on the right border of the hilum. The bile duct is ligated proximally and divided, leaving enough length for the anastomosis to the donor duct. The portal vein will be the next structure, located deeper to the artery and bile duct. If portal bypass is planned, then it can be performed at this stage. The right triangular ligament can be divided next as well as the attachments of the right lobe to the bare area.

Standard Venous Reconstruction

The left lobe of the liver is retracted up to expose the left posterior margin of the inferior vena cava (IVC). This margin is dissected from its retroperitoneal attachments starting at the level of the infrahepatic cava up to where the left

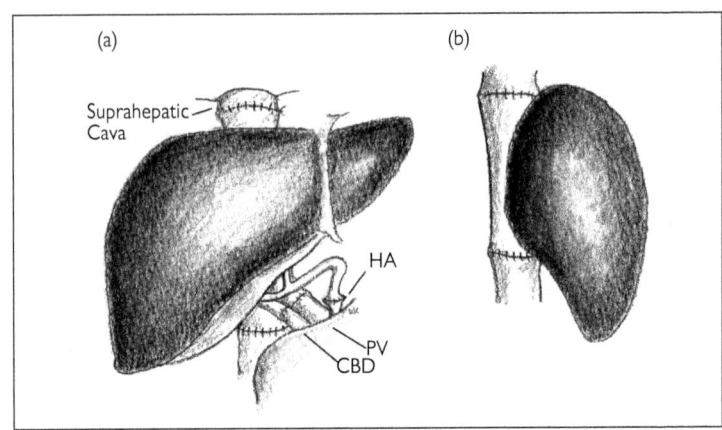

Figure 14.1. Standard caval replacement procedure for liver transplant.

phrenic vein enters the cava. The liver is then retracted to the left, and the right margin of the retro-hepatic cava is freed from its retroperitoneal tissue. Once the suprahepatic and the infrahepatic vena cava are dissected circumferentially, they are clamped, the cava is then divided, and the liver is removed along with the retrohepatic segment of cava. The suprahepatic vena cava is prepared by opening the hepatic veins into a common lumen with the IVC (Figure 14.1).

Piggyback Venous Reconstruction

The piggyback technique (Figure 14.2) involves preserving the vena cava by dissecting the liver from the anterior wall of the retrohepatic cava. The dissection involves dividing the short hepatic veins that enter the liver directly, dividing the hepato-caval ligament, and separating the caudate lobe from the caval attachments. Dissection of anterior wall of the retrohepatic cava is started inferiorly and carried superiorly to the level of the major hepatic veins. The hepatic veins are dissected and a clamp is placed across them; this is followed by division of the hepatic veins and liver explantation. After the liver is removed from the field, the bridge of tissue between the hepatic veins is divided to form a joined ostium for the suprahepatic caval anastomosis. The anastomosis between the donor suprahepatic cava and the recipient's hepatic veins is constructed in a running fashion.

Side-to-Side Cavaplasty Venous Reconstruction

The liver is mobilized as previously described, and the retrohepatic segment of cava is preserved. After the liver is removed, a "side-biting" clamp is placed on the IVC to partially occlude it. The anterior wall of the recipient cava is opened in a longitudinal fashion. The posterior wall of the donor IVC is also incised in a similar manner to match the IVC opening in the recipient. The two caval openings are anastomosed, sewing first the walls on the right side and then the

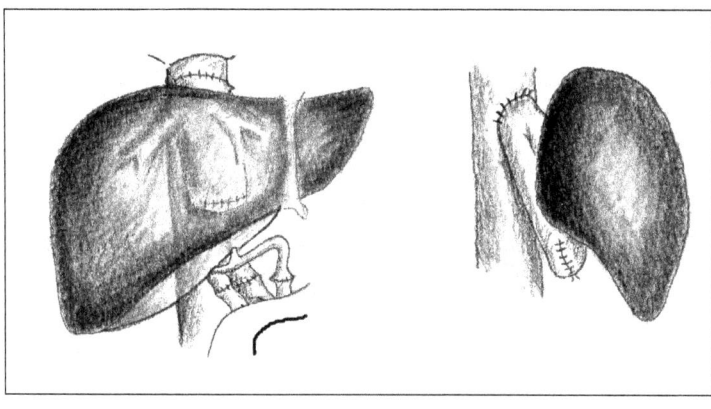

Figure 14.2. Piggyback technique for liver transplant with preservation of the recipient's native cava.

left side, both by the surgeon standing on the left side of the patient, while the surgeon on the right side assists.

Portal Reconstruction

The donor portal vein is shortened to an appropriate length. The donor portal bifurcation serves as a guide to avoid twisting or folding of the vein. If there is a significant mismatch between the donor and recipient portal veins, then the end of the smaller portal vein can be cut in a fish-mouth shape to increase the diameter. The anastomosis with the recipient portal vein is performed in an end-to-end fashion with a running 6–0 suture. It is important for the assistant surgeon not to pull too tight on the follow, as not to cinch down the suture. The ends of the prolene are tied, leaving a growth factor of 2 cm or three-fourths the size of the portal vein diameter to allow full expansion of the vein and prevent narrowing. A good size growth factor will cause some minor bleeding from the suture line that is easily corrected with an interrupted suture. The liver is generally reperfused with oxygenated blood once the portal anastomosis is completed, although some prefer to complete the arterial reconstruction before reperfusing the liver.

In the rare scenario where the recipient portal vein is unusable, the superior mesenteric vein (SMV) may be used as the inflow, using a donor iliac vein as a conduit. In this situation, the arterial reconstruction and reperfusion of the liver can be performed before the portal anastomosis. The anastomosis between the donor portal vein and the donor iliac vein conduit is performed first. Following this, the conduit is tunneled behind the stomach and anterior to the pancreas through a surgically created defect in the transverse mesocolon toward the SMV. A side-occluding clamp is placed on the SMV, and the anastomosis is performed in an end-to-side fashion.

Arterial Reconstruction

The goal of the arterial reconstruction is to re-establish optimal arterial flow by selecting healthy vessels and adequately matched size arteries and performing an anastomosis with vessels of good diameter. For routine cases with standard anatomy, a patch of the donor's hepatic artery with a branch (gastroduodenal artery or the splenic artery) is sewn to the recipient's common hepatic artery or to a branch patch. If the donor's common hepatic artery or arterial branch patch are of small caliber, then the celiac trunk with a Carrel patch of donor aorta could be used for the anastomosis to the recipient. However, when using the celiac for the anastomosis, one needs to ensure that the artery lays without significant folding.

Because of the variable hepatic arterial anatomy, the surgeon may be presented with different scenarios for reconstruction. The donor's gastroduodenal or splenic artery can be used to establish arterial continuity with a donor accessory right or left hepatic artery, if present. If the recipient has a dominant replaced right hepatic artery, then the main arterial anastomosis should be done to this vessel using the donor's hepatic artery or celiac artery.

In the setting where the recipient has no acceptable hepatic artery to which the donor vessel can be anastomosed, a donor iliac artery can be used for conduit. For this procedure, the abdominal aorta just above the inferior mesenteric artery is exposed. The aorta is side-occluded, and the iliac conduit is sewn end to side. The conduit is then tunneled through the transverse mesocolon, behind and stomach and anterior to the pancreas to the hepatic hilum, where it is anastomosed end to end to the donor common hepatic artery or a branch patch of the hepatic artery.

Biliary Reconstruction

The gallbladder is removed, if not done so already on the back table. Depending on the patient's anatomy and underlying disease, the options for biliary anastomosis include:

choledocho-choledochostomy (duct to duct)
choledocho-duodenostomy
choledocho-jejunostomy

Traditionally the donor common bile duct (CBD) is sewn in an end-to-end fashion to the recipient CBD (choledocho-choledochostomy or duct-to-duct anastomosis). If the recipient's common bile duct cannot be used (e.g., sclerosing cholangitis), then the biliary reconstruction can be done as a choledocho-jejunostomy. If the recipients' CBD is unusable and mobilizing a jejunal roux limb for a choledocho-jejunostomy is not a safe option because of extensive adhesions, then the duodenum can be mobilized and brought up to the hepatic hilum to perform a choledocho-duodenostomy.

Internal or external biliary stents can be placed across the biliary anastomosis. The stent should be secured with absorbable suture to the bowel wall mucosa to prevent it from coming out too soon. The external stent is placed using a Witzel technique to bring it out of the bowel lumen and through the abdominal wall. The Witzel technique helps to prevent bile leaks when the biliary stent is removed 4 to 6 weeks later. The advantage of having an external stent is the ease with which interrogation of the biliary anastomosis and biliary tree can be performed in the postoperative period.

Living Donor Liver Procedure

A partial hepatectomy in an otherwise healthy donor is a major undertaking. Surgeons involved in living donor liver procedures must have an extensive knowledge of the intrahepatic as well as the extrahepatic anatomy; familiarity with parenchymal transection techniques and reconstruction of the biliary and vascular system on the recipient side is necessary. In addition to the demanding technical aspect of this procedure, good clinical judgment in the pre-operative setting is of utmost importance to assure that the appropriate candidates for donation are selected. This includes assessing the medical fitness of the individual, radiological testing to evaluate the liver anatomy, and a psychosocial interview. Donor and recipients are routinely discussed in a multidisciplinary conference, and approval of all the different specialties involved is necessary prior to proceeding with the operation.

Adult Recipient

Donor Surgery: Right Lobectomy

The falciform ligament and the right triangular ligament are divided. The liver is mobilized to the left by dividing the lateral attachments of the right lobe to the bare area; at this point, the right lateral aspect of the retrohepatic cava should be visible. The multiple small tributaries from the right lobe to the vena cava are ligated and divided. Any branch 0.5 cm or larger should be preserved for potential later reconstruction on the recipient side. The dissection of the lateral aspect of the cava is carried up toward the right hepatic vein. The hepatocaval ligament will be encountered inferior and to the right in relation to the right hepatic vein. This ligament may contain a vein; therefore, it is always suture ligated and divided. At this stage, one can proceed to dissect and encircle the right hepatic vein with umbilical tape.

The hilar plate is taken down and the common hepatic duct bifurcation identified. The right hepatic artery, which is usually found to the right of the common bile duct is carefully dissected. Next, the right lateral aspect of the hepatoduodenal ligament is dissected, staying posterior to the right hepatic artery to identify the portal vein and the right portal branch. The right portal vein should be dissected circumferentially and the bifurcation area to the left portal vein identified. Small branches to the caudate lobe from the right portal vein, if present, should be ligated and divided. With all the hilar structures isolated, one can proceed to perform a cholangiogram to delineate the biliary tree anatomy and safely transect the common bile duct. Depending on the biliary anatomy, one may have more than one bile duct to reconstruct after the transection, such as in the case of a right sectoral duct draining into the left duct. The right hepatic duct should be transected at a point, where there would be a sufficient stump left to oversew without impinging on the lumen of the left hepatic duct. An intra-operative ultrasound is performed to identify the middle hepatic vein and any significant tributary from segments V and VIII. The parenchymal transection will be carried to the right of the middle hepatic vein. An Umbilical tape is passed through the junction of the right and middle hepatic veins, behind the right lobe of the liver and anterior to the right hepatic artery, then placed under some light tension to help guide the plane of parenchymal transection. The parenchymal transection is performed with electrocautery for the first few millimeters of parenchyma. Further division of the parenchyma should be done with any of the different devices available for hepatic transection and/or with the clamp-crush technique. Any large tributaries (≥5 mm) draining to the middle hepatic vein should be marked for later reconstruction on the recipient side. Once the parenchymal transection is completed, the graft is only attached by the vascular structures and the biliary duct (Figure 14.3). At this point the right hepatic duct is divided, and if the recipient team is ready, then one may proceed to divide the hepatic artery, followed by the portal vein and the right hepatic vein last. The right hepatic artery can be divided between clamps. A vascular stapler can be used for the right portal vein, ensuring that the device fires in an anterior-to-posterior manner so as to not narrow the left portal vein. The right hepatic vein is divided with a laparoscopic vascular stapler. The graft is passed to the recipient team. Careful hemostasis of the cut-edge of the liver is done. The falciform ligament is reattached using a running suture to stabilize the left lobe. A drain may be placed, depending on the surgeon's preference. The incision is then closed.

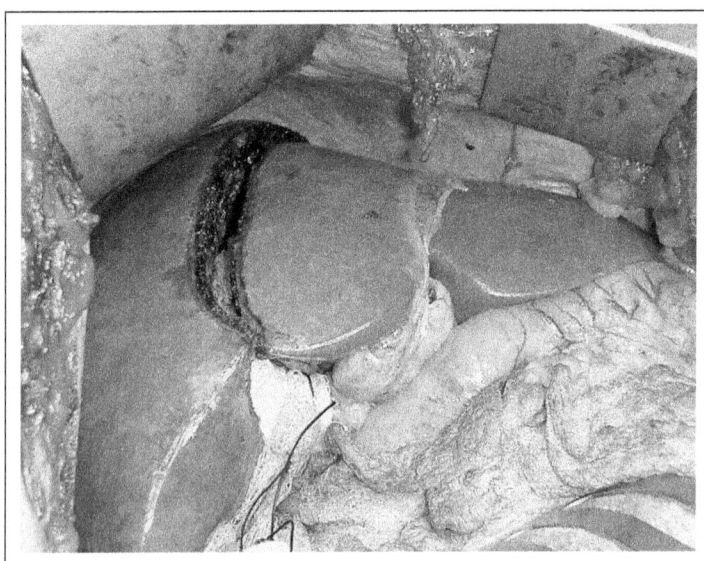

Figure 14.3. Intra-operative photo showing transection of hepatic parenchyma just before removing the right lobe graft.

Donor Surgery: Left Lobectomy

The principles are similar to those for right lobectomy. The falciform ligament and left triangular ligaments are taken down. The suprahepatic cava is dissected anteriorly. The gastrohepatic ligament is opened with careful attention for a possible replaced or accessory left hepatic artery coming from the left gastric artery. Next, a cholecystectomy and cannulation of the cystic duct for an intra-operative cholangiogram is performed. Attention can then be turned to dissection of the hilar structures. The left hepatic duct, left hepatic artery, and left portal vein are dissected, usually in this order. After the hilar structures are isolated, the left lobe is lifted up toward the right side, and dissection is continued along the left lateral aspect of the retrohepatic vena cava up to the level of the insertion of the left hepatic vein. The venous branches draining directly into the cava from the left lobe are ligated and divided. After this retrohepatic dissection is completed, one should to isolate the left and middle hepatic veins. At this stage, an intra-operative cholangiogram is performed to confirm the biliary anatomy and safely proceed with division of the left biliary duct. Following this, an intra-operative ultrasound is used to identify the middle hepatic vein and any major tributaries. The parenchymal transection for the left lobectomy will be carried just to the right of this vein. Again, an umbilical tape is passed behind the left lobe and anterior to the hilar structures for the "liver-hanging" maneuver to guide the hepatic transection. Once the parenchymal transection is completed, attention is turned to the vascular structures. The left hepatic artery is clamped and divided, followed by the left portal branch, and finally the confluence of the middle and left hepatic veins. During division of the hepatic veins, care must be taken to avoid encroachment of the donor's vasculature after sewing or ligation.

Recipient Surgery

A standard cava-preserving hepatectomy is performed. For the venous reconstruction, the donor's right hepatic vein is anastomosed to the orifice of the recipient's right hepatic vein, with an extension along the anterior wall of the recipient's cava, if necessary, to ensure adequate outflow. In cases of a left lobe graft, the left and middle hepatic veins are anastomosed to the orifice of the left hepatic and middle hepatic veins, respectively, on the donor side with an extension to the recipient's right hepatic vein or to the anterior wall of the cava, when necessary. Notably, it is important to keep the donor's hepatic vein short to avoid torsion. Significant venous tributaries previously reconstructed during the back table procedure are anastomosed at this time. The venous branches can be anastomosed directly to the anterior wall of the cava or to one of the orifices of the recipient's suprahepatic veins. Options for conduits for venous reconstruction of any large tributary are cryopreserved veins or the recipient's saphenous femoral vein. The donor's right or left portal vein is anastomosed to the corresponding recipient's portal vein or the main portal vein. Portal vein alignment is key when doing this reconstruction. In the setting of two portal vein branches to the graft (most commonly a separate right anterior and right posterior portal branch with a right lobe graft), the reconstruction can be done with a y-graft from a cryopreserved iliac vein or to the recipient's left and right portal vein as long as the alignment permits. After the hepatic vein and portal vein anastomosis are completed, the graft can be flushed. For the hepatic artery reconstruction, it is helpful to have divided the hepatic artery as proximal to the liver as possible on the recipient side to have options for reconstruction in the setting of one or multiple arteries. The arterial anastomosis is completed in an interrupted fashion with a 7–0 or 8–0 Prolene. The bile duct can be completed as a duct-to-duct anastomosis or as a roux-en-y loop jejunostomy. To perform a duct-to-duct anastomosis, it is important to divide the recipient's bile duct high in the hepatic hilum; the length may permit a tension-free anastomosis and provide the right, left, and cystic bile ducts as options for reconstruction in the setting of multiple donor bile ducts. The bile duct anastomosis is usually completed over an internal stent. A choledocho-jejunal anastomosis is also an option, even in the setting of one or more donor bile ducts. All biliary anastomosis should be fashioned tension-free and should be checked for leaks at their completion. Closed suction drains are placed in the dependent areas as well as the cut edge of the graft.

Deceased Donor Split Liver Procedure

The splitting of a deceased donor liver organ can be achieved in two ways. In the *in situ* technique the splitting is done as part of the "warm" dissection during a multi-organ procurement procedure. In the *ex situ* technique, the donor organ is retrieved and then split on the back table in a cold preservation solution.

Prior to starting a split liver transplant (SLT), the standard procedures of abdominal organ procurement, including sternotomy, supraceliac, and infrarenal aortic dissection as well as cannulation of the inferior mesenteric vein, should be completed such that if the donor were to become unstable, the SLT could be aborted with rapid progression to aortic cannulation, aortic cross-clamping, suprahepatic cava venting, and organ cold perfusion.

Extended Right/Left Lateral Segment Split (Adult/Pediatric Recipients)

The operation starts by taking down the falciform ligament all the way up to the diaphragm, followed by the left triangular ligament. The left hepatic vein is dissected and encircled with a vessel loop. In some cases, the bifurcation of the left and middle hepatic vein occurs within the liver parenchyma, and control of the left hepatic vein may not be obtained until after some degree of hepatic transection. After the left hepatic vein is isolated, attention is turned to the left hilar plate. The goal at this step is to dissect the left hepatic artery and left portal vein and continue dissection up toward the umbilical fissure. Ideally, the segment IV artery that branches from the left hepatic artery is preserved. If the segment IV artery is of significant diameter and it branches high on the left hepatic artery, then it should be reconstructed, usually by anastomosing it to the recipient's gastroduodenal artery. The portal vein at this level has several small branches to segment IV that must be divided. After completion of this dissection, the left hilar plate should lay open. After the hilar structures are isolated, the lateral limb of the vessel loop around the left hepatic vein can be passed anterior to the arterial and portal bifurcation, and it may be placed on slight tension to guide the transection line in the angle between the left and middle hepatic veins.

In the *ex situ* technique, the whole organ is removed using standard cadaveric donor procurements procedures, and the parenchyma is transected on the back table using a sharp blade. At the end of the transection, the two grafts are only connected by the hilar plate. This is also transected sharply.

In the *in situ* technique, the parenchymal transection is completed using traditional liver surgery techniques. After the transection is completed, the surgeon has two options for cold perfusion. The vessels can be clamped and divided, and the left lateral segment can be removed and flushed on the back table, leaving perfusion of the extended right lobe with the rest of the organs *in situ*. This allows for potential transplantation of the left graft earlier. The second option is to perfuse both grafts *in situ* and then separate the vasculature of the grafts on the back table.

Full Right/Full Left Split (Adult/Adult Recipients)

The vascular control and the parenchymal transection technique is essentially the same for right lobe living donation. However, there are few differences and key points to keep in mind. It must be recognized that more liver tissue is needed in deceased donor liver transplantation than in living donor transplantation. This results from the worse condition of deceased donor grafts in general and the longer ischemia times. One of the strategies to minimize ischemia times is to do most of the dissection in situ. As opposed to living donation, in deceased donors, the vena cava can be procured providing large venous cuffs along with the grafts, including the minor hepatic veins of the caudate lobe, which can be important hepatic mass for the left lobe.

Selected References

Neuhaus P, Blumhardt G, Bechstein WO, Steffen R, Platz KP, & Keck H. Technique and results of biliary reconstruction using side-to-side choledocholedochostomy in 300 orthotopic liver transplants. *Ann Surg.* 1994;219(4):426–434.

Trotter JF, Wachs M, Everson GT, & Kam I. Adult-to-adult transplantation of the right hepatic lobe from a living donor. *N Engl J Med.* 2002;346(14):1074–1082.

Chapter 15

Graft Dysfunction and Technical Complications After Liver Transplant

Abhideep Chaudhary and Abhinav Humar

Introduction

The risk of developing postoperative complications is related to the patient's preoperative condition, the quality of the donor liver, the quality of the donor and recipient procedure, initial graft function, and perioperative anesthetic and intensive care management. Complications occurring early after transplant are mainly related to the technical aspects of the procedure or functional issues with the graft. Surgical complications related directly to the operation include post-operative hemorrhage and anastomotic complications (vascular and/or biliary). Graft rejection is also an important cause of graft dysfunction, which can occur both early and late post-transplant.

Graft Dysfunction

The differential diagnosis of liver transplant dysfunction depends on the time at which it occurs. Abnormal liver tests soon after transplantation may reflect functional or technical problems, such as primary graft nonfunction, ischemia reperfusion injury, vascular or biliary complication, or may even be secondary to shock and sepsis.

Primary Nonfunction

Primary nonfunction (PNF) is a devastating complication seen in less than 5% of transplants, with a mortality rate of more than 80% without a retransplant. It reflects poor or no hepatic function from the time of the transplant procedure. The cause of PNF is unknown, but several donor factors like advanced age, increased fat content of the donor liver, longer donor hospital stay before organ procurement, prolonged cold ischemia (>18 hours), and reduced-sized grafts may predict development of this syndrome.

Early prediction of PNF is valuable in identifying patients that will need a retransplant. It is also important to rule out conditions that may mimic PNF such as hepatic artery thrombosis, hyper-acute rejection, and severe infection. Primary nonfunction should be considered in recipients who do not regain consciousness or who have increasing renal dysfunction, continued hemodynamic instability, increasing prothrombin time, or persistent hypoglycemia. An AST (aspartate aminotransferase) greater than 5000 IU/L, Factor VIII less than 60% of normal, PT greater than 20 seconds at 4 to 6 hours post-reperfusion, in association with poor bile production, may all suggest PNF.

Unfortunately, no medical treatment is effective for PNF. Intravenous prostaglandin E1 (PGE1) has some useful effect, but further evaluation is necessary. Its mechanism of action is presumably a vasodilatory effect on the splanchnic circulation, resulting in enhanced blood flow to the new liver. Recipients with suspected PNF should probably be started on a continuous infusion and listed for an urgent retransplant. The starting dose is 0.005 µg/kg/min, which is increased, as tolerated per blood pressure measurements, to a maximum of 0.03 µg/kg/min. Ultimately, such recipients do better with a retransplant. However, if a retransplant is to positively influence outcome, then it must be done before multi-organ failure develops. In one series of 15 liver recipients with PNF, all those who sustained organ failure in four or more systems died despite a retransplant.

Reperfusion Injury

The ischemia reperfusion injury (IRI), also known as preservation injury, is an important cause of early graft dysfunction and has a major impact on success of liver transplantation. Ischemia reperfusion injury is defined as the phenomenon whereby cellular damage in a hypoxic organ is accentuated following the restoration of oxygen delivery.

In solid organ transplantation, graft damage subsequent to IRI may be responsible for delayed graft function or, in extreme cases, PNF. Some degree of hepatic IRI is inevitable in liver transplantation and its etiology is of multifactorial origin.

Various risk factors for development of IRI or graft dysfunction have been identified, including donor age older than 60 years, macrovesicular steatosis, high inotropic drug use, hypernatremia, prolonged intensive care stays, donation after cardiac death, prolonged cold ischemia time, and long anhepatic phase in the recipient.

Ischemia reperfusion injury is suspected based on the laboratory abnormalities, including prolonged hyperbilirubinemia in a recipient with the risk factors mentioned above, and diagnosis can be confirmed by liver biopsy. Ischemia reperfusion injuries usually resolve in 2 to 4 weeks, but severe IRI is associated with increased morbidity, graft loss, and mortality.

Vascular Complications

The incidence of vascular complications after liver transplant is 5% to 10%. Thrombosis is the most common early event; stenosis, dissection, and pseudo-aneurysm formation are less common. Any of the vascular anastomoses may be involved, but the hepatic artery is most common.

Hepatic Artery Thrombosis

Hepatic artery thrombosis (HAT) is the most common vascular complication after liver transplant and has a reported incidence of 3% to 5% in adults and about 5% to 8% in children. Several risk factors have been reported for early HAT, including retransplantation, use of arterial conduits, prolonged operation and cold ischemic times, low recipient weight, severe rejection, variant arterial anatomy, and low-volume transplantation centers. Technical factors that disturb laminar flow of the blood in the arteries (such as intimal dissection, tension on the anastomosis, and kinking of the artery) are also implicated in the development of HAT. Thrombosis rates are higher after split-liver and living related transplants because of the smaller caliber of vessels and the complex arterial reconstruction required.

After HAT, liver recipients may be asymptomatic or may have severe liver failure secondary to extensive necrosis, depending on the interval between transplant and the onset of HAT. Those with thrombosis early post-operatively, especially adults, have the most dramatic signs and symptoms: marked elevation of serum transaminase levels, septic shock, encephalopathy, and overall rapid deterioration. Ultrasound with Doppler evaluation is the initial investigation of choice, with more than 90% sensitivity and specificity (Fig. 15.1). Diagnosis can be confirmed by angiography (Fig. 15.1). Prompt re-exploration with thrombectomy and revision of the anastomoses is indicated if the diagnosis is made early. If hepatic necrosis is extensive, then a retransplant is indicated. Computed tomography or MRI scans may be helpful in determining the extent of necrosis. Most centers use routine protocol Doppler ultrasound post-transplant, but some centers—including ours—use implantable Doppler probes performing continuous flow monitoring in patients with high risk for development of HAT.

Hepatic artery thrombosis may also present in a less dramatic fashion. The donor bile duct receives its blood supply from the hepatic artery. Thrombosis may therefore render the common bile duct ischemic, resulting in a localized or diffuse bile leak from the anastomosis, intrahepatic abscess, cholangitis and sepsis, or more chronically a diffuse biliary stricture. (Fig. 15.2). These groups of patients are best treated by retransplant, but until an organ becomes available, they can be managed with endoscopic retrograde cholangiopancreatography (ERCP) and stent placement or percutaneous transhepatic cholioangiography (PTC) and antibiotics.

Late thrombosis may be asymptomatic, especially in children, because of the presence of collaterals along the biliary anastomosis, which provide sufficient arterial inflow. These patients can be followed with expectant management based on their symptoms.

The outcome of patients with HAT depends on timing of diagnosis and severity of presentation. With prompt re-exploration, thrombectomy, and revision of the anastomoses, graft salvage can be achieved in 10% to 25% cases (with higher

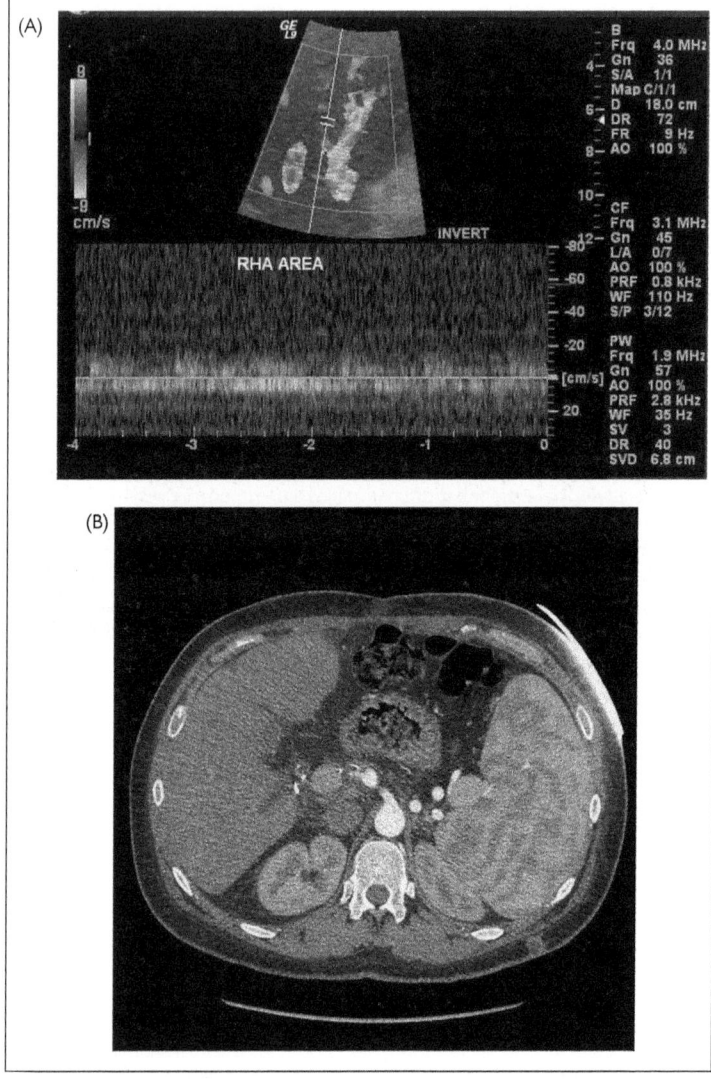

Figure 15.1. Hepatic artery thrombosis. **(A)** Absent flow in hepatic artery as no signal on spectral Doppler. **(B)** Computed tomography angiogram demonstrating HAT. **(C)** Reconstructed computed tomography angiogram demonstrating HAT. **(D)** Angiogram showing flow in celiac trunk and splenic artery but no flow in hepatic artery.

(C)

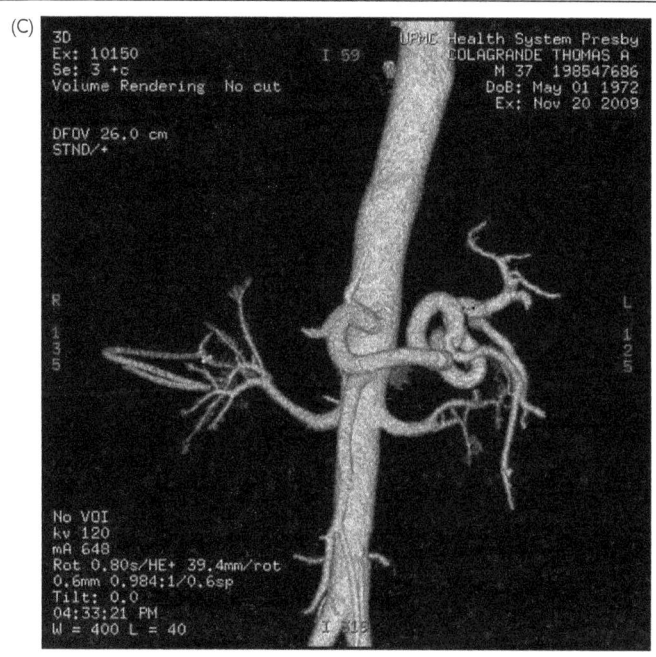

(D)

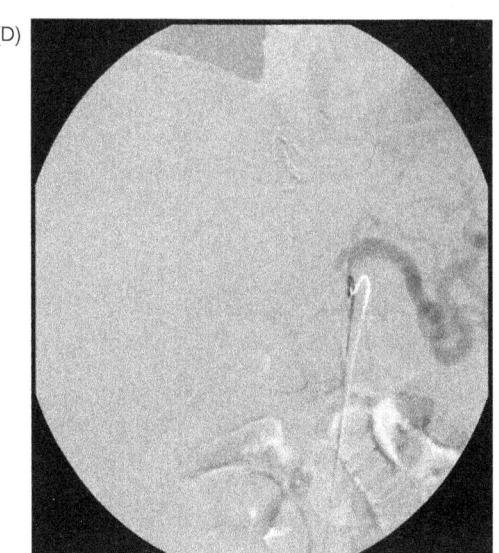

Figure 15.1. (*Continued*)

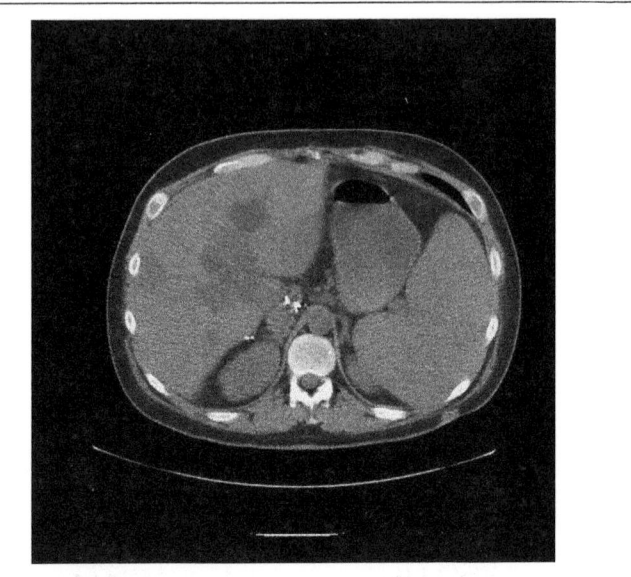

Figure 15.2. Computed tomography demonstrating intrahepatic biliary ductal dilatation with central ill-defined biloma in a patient with late HAT.

salvage rates in HAT diagnosed with screening ultrasound Doppler). Eventually 50% to 70% patients with HAT require retransplant, and despite treatment measures, HAT is associated with a mortality rate of 10% to 30%.

Hepatic Artery Stenosis

Hepatic artery stenosis (HAS), often seen at the site of anastomosis, occurs in about 10% of cases. This can lead to biliary ischemia and hepatic dysfunction and, if severe, can progress to thrombosis. Routine Doppler ultrasonography is a sensitive method for diagnosis with findings of low resistive index and high systolic acceleration time; celiac angiography can be done to confirm the diagnosis.

Celiac artery stenosis may be seen because of Medial Arcuate Ligament syndrome or atherosclerotic changes, which can be treated by surgical division of the arcuate ligament or an aortohepatic graft interposition. Interventional treatment by percutaneous transluminal angioplasty is used in the management of stenotic lesions after liver transplantation, often in combination with stents (Fig. 15.3).

Portal Vein Thrombosis and Stenosis

Portal vein thrombosis (PVT) is far less frequent (compared with the hepatic artery), occurring in fewer than 2% of recipients. It may be related to a technical factor such as narrowing of the anastomosis or excessive length of the portal

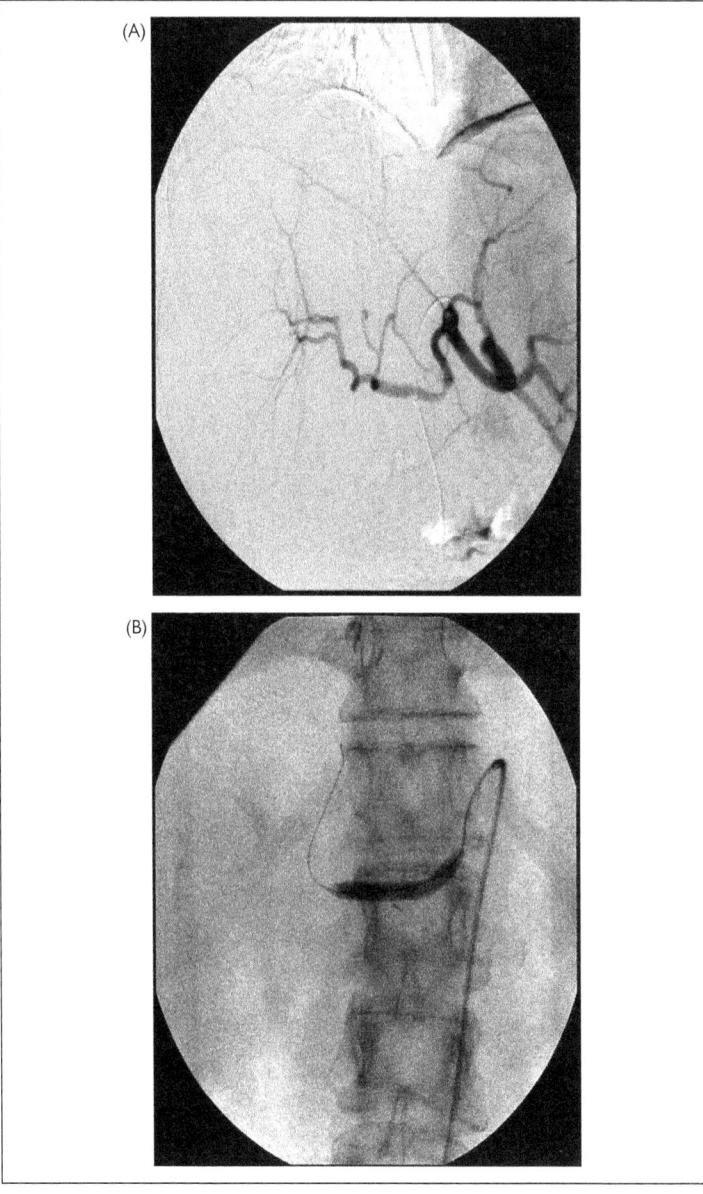

Figure 15.3. Hepatic artery stenosis. Angiogram demonstrating **(A)** HAS, **(B)** dilatation, and **(C)** post-dilatation.

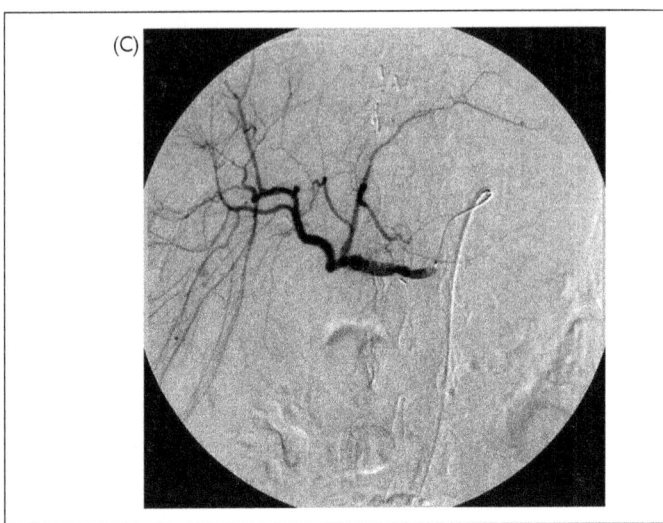

(C)

Figure 15.3. (*Continued*)

vein with kinking. Recipients who require a venous conduit secondary to underlying PVT are at higher risk for PVT. Other risk factors include pretransplant portosystemic shunt, previous splenectomy, or hypercoagulable state. Incidence of PVT is slightly higher in pediatric liver transplant recipients, especially in infants and children with biliary atresia. Early post-operatively, PVT may result in severe liver dysfunction. Tense ascites and variceal bleeding may be seen secondary to acutely elevated portal and mesenteric venous pressures. If these symptoms develop post-operatively, then urgent ultrasound with Doppler evaluation is performed to assess the patency of the portal vein (Fig. 15.4). If the diagnosis is made early, then operative thrombectomy and revision of the anastomosis may be successful, but patients with severe liver dysfunction may require emergent retransplant. Portal vein thrombosis can also be managed nonsurgically by percutaneous portal vein thrombolysis, systemic anticoagulation, and stenting. If thrombosis occurs late, then liver function is usually preserved because of the presence of collaterals. In these cases, a retransplant is often not necessary; management is conservative with systemic anticoagulation, and attention diverted toward relieving the left-sided portal hypertension.

Portal vein stenosis (PVS) is an uncommon complication occurring in 1% to 2% of recipients and is usually secondary to the same technical factors as mentioned for PVT above. Portal vein stenosis is suspected in patients with signs of elevated portal pressure or diagnosed on routine Doppler ultrasound. Ultrasound findings of PVS include focal narrowing of the portal vein, elevated anastomotic velocities greater than 150 cm/s, or a ratio greater than 4:1 between the anastomotic and pre-anastomotic velocities (Fig.15.5).

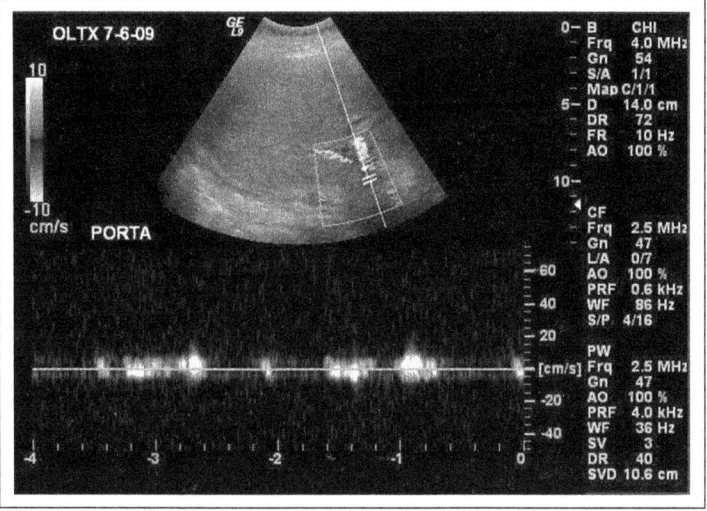

Figure 15.4. Portal vein thrombosis. Absent flow in portal vein as no signal on spectral Doppler.

Portal vein stenosis can be treated with percutaneous balloon dilatation (Fig. 15.5) or by surgical revision of the anastomosis.

Hepatic Vein/Caval Complications

Complications of the hepatic veins (such as thrombosis and stenosis) are rare, with an incidence of less than 1% in deceased donor liver transplant and 1% to 10% in live donor liver transplant. Recurrence of Budd-Chiari syndrome and technical factors such as narrowing of the anastomosis are the most common causes. Other causes that are more specific to piggyback technique or live donor transplant include torsion or compression of the veins. The risk of thrombosis is higher in recipients of a left lateral segment, either from a living donor or as part of a split-liver graft. This segment may be quite mobile and, if not properly aligned, may twist, resulting in outflow obstruction. Presentation is usually with massive ascites, graft dysfunction, and occasionally edema or renal insufficiency. Again, Doppler ultrasound will usually demonstrate the problem. On ultrasound, the normal hepatic vein and inferior vena cava (IVC) waveform is triphasic, but significant caval stenosis may result in reversed flow or absence of phasicity in the hepatic veins and the infrahepatic IVC. The findings can be confirmed by venocavogram, and a fixed pressure gradient of more than 10 mmHg is confirmatory.

Balloon dilatation with or without stent placement has been successful for hepatic vein/caval stenosis (Fig. 15.6). If this approach is not successful, then direct surgical approaches or retransplantation will be required for patients with

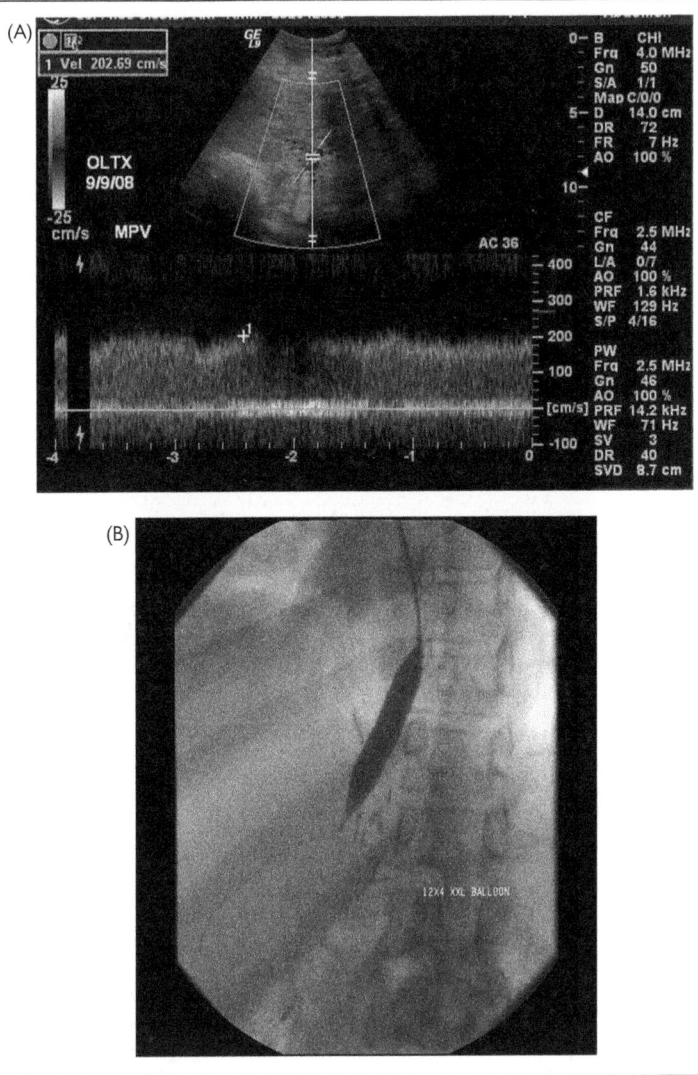

Figure 15.5. Portal vein stenosis. **(A)** Spectral Doppler showing increased velocity in portal vein. **(B)** Portal venogram demonstrating stenosis at portal venous anastomosis site. **(C)** Balloon dilatation of stenotic region. **(D)** Demonstrating resolution of portal vein stenosis.

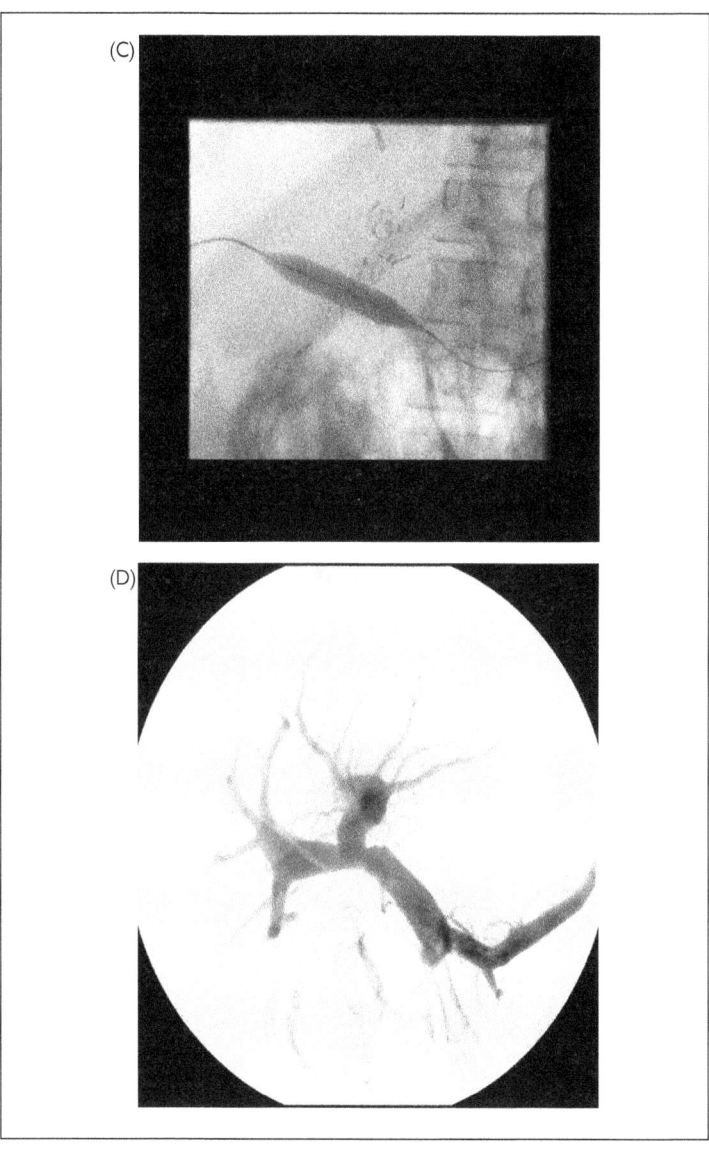

Figure 15.5. (*Continued*)

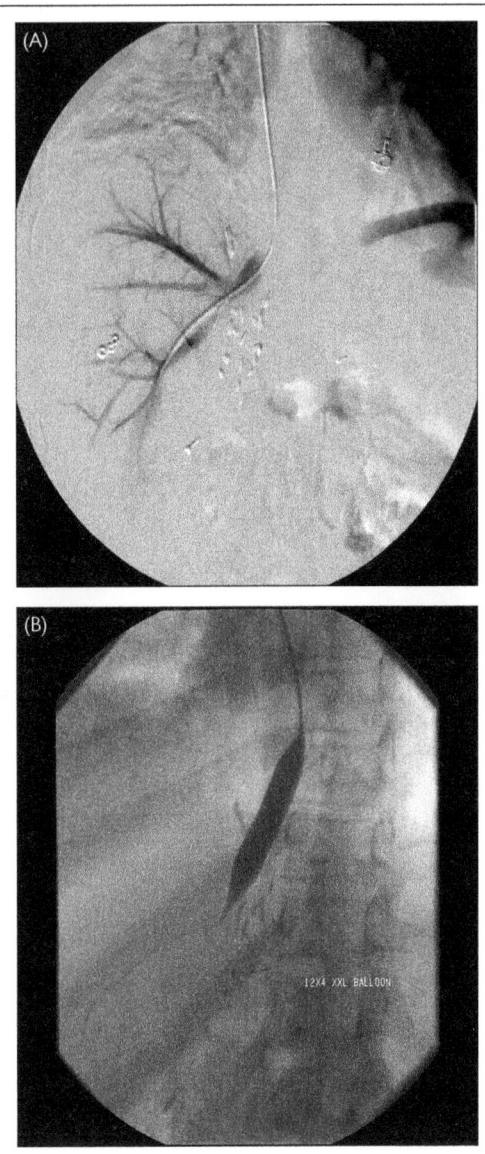

Figure 15.6. Hepatic vein stenosis. Venocavogram demonstrating **(A)** stenosis at piggyback hepatic venous anastomosis site; **(B)** balloon dilatation of stenotic region; and **(C)** resolution of stenosis.

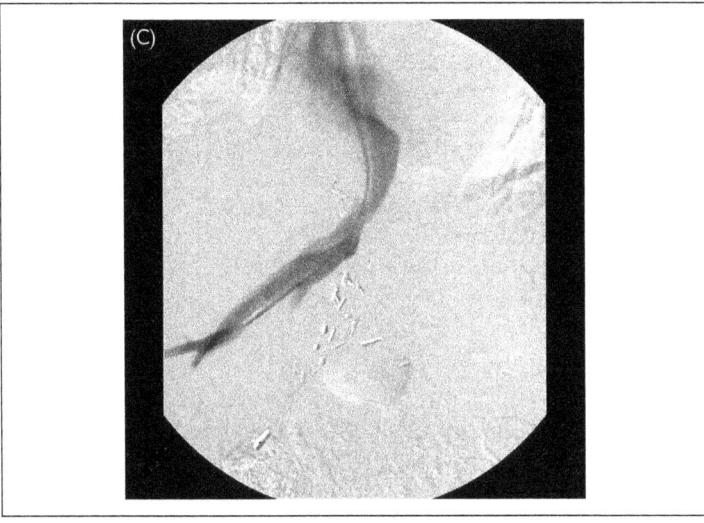

Figure 15.6. (*Continued*)

suprahepatic vena caval obstruction. Early anticoagulation is required to prevent recurrence of Budd-Chiari syndrome. Urgent retransplantation is required only in rare cases, where the thrombosis of the hepatic veins completely or near completely obstructs the vena cava.

Biliary Complications

Complications of the biliary system continue to be common after liver transplantation. Biliary complications occur in 10% to 15% of all patients receiving a full-size graft. The incidence in living donor, split-, or reduced-size liver transplantations has been reported in a range of 15% to 30%, with an associated mortality of less than 5%. Complications may result from devascularization of the bile duct at the hilar dissection, failure to recognize anomalies of the biliary tree, technically challenging biliary reconstruction (small-size ducts, multiple ducts), and biliary leaks from the cut surface in a partial liver transplant.

Biliary leaks and strictures are the most common biliary complications, but ampullary stenosis or dysfunction, hemobilia, and biliary obstruction from cystic duct mucocele, stones, sludge, or casts have also been reported. The majority of biliary complications occur within the first 3 months after transplant. Timing will often determine type and clinical outcome of the complication.

Bile Leak

Most bile leaks occur within the first 30 days post-transplant. Bile leak may be anastomotic or non-anastomotic. In whole-liver transplant recipients, biliary leaks occur most commonly at the anastomotic site. The area around the anastomosis has the most tenuous blood supply: Both the donor common bile duct (CBD) and the recipient portion of the CBD are supplied by end arteries. Excessive dissection or cauterization around the donor or recipient CBD can further disrupt the blood supply, leading to ischemic complications. Another important cause of biliary tract complications is HAT: The donor CBD receives its blood supply from the hepatic artery. With any biliary tract complication, the hepatic artery should be carefully assessed to document patency. Other causes of leaks include poorly placed sutures, excessive number of sutures, and tension on the anastomosis. Non-anastomotic leaks such as those occurring at the T-tube insertion site may be observed. Most centers have abandoned the use of external T-tube stents because a leak may occur from the T-tube site in up to 33% cases when it is removed. With partial transplants, the cut surface of the liver represents the most common site for a bile leak occurring in up to 20% cases. Less frequently, biliary leaks may occur later than 3 months after transplantation and are usually caused by either persistence of early complications or a late HAT.

Clinical symptoms of a bile leak include fever, abdominal pain, and peritoneal irritation. Bile in the abdominal drains is highly suspicious for a leak, but absence of bile in the drains does not preclude the diagnosis. Blood tests may demonstrate an elevation of the white blood cell count, bilirubin, and alkaline phosphatase; unfortunately, no laboratory test is pathognomonic. Ultrasound may demonstrate a fluid collection, but often cholangiography is required for diagnosis. This is simple to perform if an external biliary stent is in place. In the absence of an external stent, options include magnetic resonance cholangiography (MRC), endoscopic retrograde cholangiography (ERC), or PTC (Fig. 15.7).

Bile leaks occurring immediately after transplant are best treated by surgical exploration. The anastomosis is revised, or for small leaks, additional sutures are placed at the leak site. If there is undue tension in recipients with a duct-to-duct anastomosis, then the biliary anastomosis is converted to a choledochojejunostomy.

The increasing popularity of treating nontransplant biliary leaks with endoscopically placed stents has led to their use for transplant-related leaks. Anastomotic leaks can be successfully treated in more than 90% without surgery with endoscopic stenting, if the leak is localized without major biliary extravasion (Fig. 15.7).

If the anastomosis is severely disrupted, or biliary extravasation is substantial, then surgical revision is required. Leakage from the T-tube site can be managed by opening the T-tube to divert bile flow or responds to endoscopic stent placement. In patients with reduced-size transplantation or LDLT leaks may occur from the cut surface. These leaks can be managed by ERC and sphincterotomy to reduce the intraductal pressure and to achieve optimal biliary flow, or a temporary percutaneous drainage is required in cases of bilioenteric anastomosis. Late biliary leaks may be accompanied by strictures following ischemic damage.

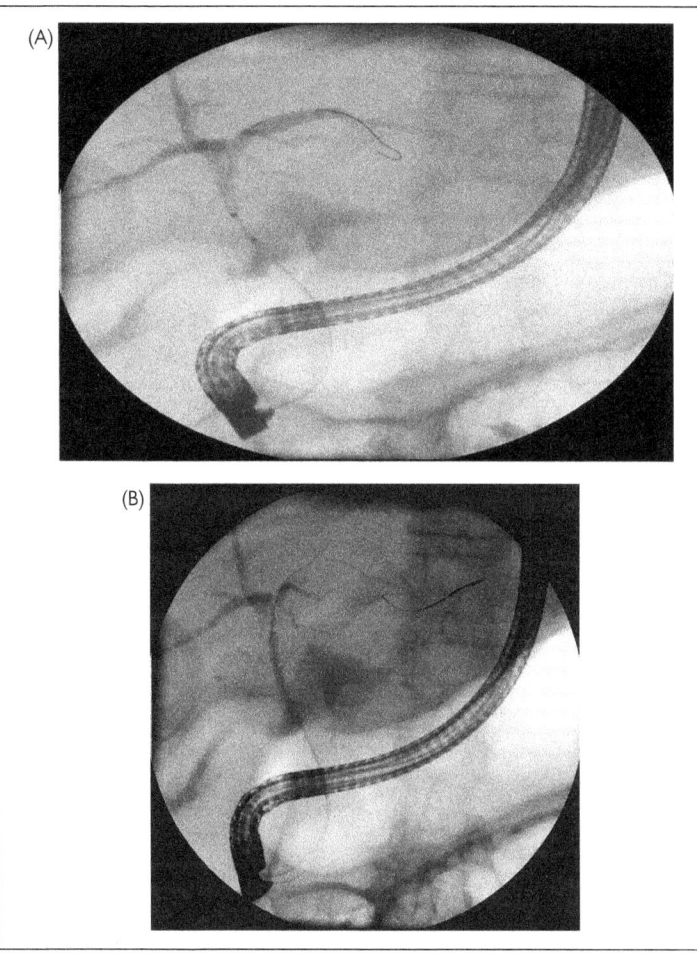

Figure 15.7. Endoscopic retrograde cholangiography demonstrating **(A)** anastomotic bile leak and **(B)** stenting.

Cases with associated intra-abdominal bile collection (biloma) should be treated by percutaneous ultrasound-guided or CT-guided drainage.

Biliary Stricture

Biliary strictures account for one-third of biliary complications after liver transplant and occur later in the post-operative period. It is most common at the anastomotic site and is likely related to local ischemia and fibrosis or technical error. According to some series of whole-organ transplant, anastomotic strictures are reported to be more common after hepaticojejunostomy than after direct duct-to-duct anastomosis. Non-anastomotic strictures often are in the hilar region, but diffuse intrahepatic manifestations are also observed and usually have a worse prognosis; they are associated with HAT or HAS, prolonged cold ischemic times, and ABO-incompatible donors.

Patients with biliary stricture usually present with cholestasis (increased bilirubin, alkaline phosphatase, and gamma-glutamyl transferase) or cholangitis, or both. Leukocytosis, fever, and right upper quadrant pain may often be absent in the case of cholangitis. Ultrasound can be misleading in making the diagnosis, because ductal dilatation may not be seen; however, it is still a crucial test to exclude potential hepatic arterial flow complications (which is a potential cause of bile duct stricture). Cholangiography (T-tube cholangiography, ERC, MRC, or PTC, depending on the type of BD reconstruction performed) is always necessary for diagnosis of BD stricture (Figs. 15.8 and 15.9).

The treatment for anastomotic and common bile duct stricture is usually not operative but, rather, by percutaneous or endoscopic internal balloon dilatation and stent placement across the site of stricture (Figs. 15.8 and 15.9). This has a long-term success rate of more than 50% to 70%. If these initial options fail, then surgical revision is required. The non-anastomotic strictures resulting from HAT have a much worse prognosis, and a nonsurgical interventional treatment should be considered to bridge the patient to liver retransplantation as mentioned previously. In patients with donor hepatic duct strictures not related to HAT, repeated endoscopic or percutaneous interventions are needed. Surgical revision with roux-en-Y anastomosis is reserved for patients in whom balloon dilatation and stenting are unsuccessful. Treatment of diffuse intrahepatic strictures is more difficult. Balloon dilatation and stenting of dominant strictures may provide temporary palliation, but in advanced biliary disease, retransplantation is required.

Rejection

Acute rejection is very common after a liver transplant; 20% to 30% of recipients will have at least one bout at some point post-transplant, but only 5% to 10% of liver transplant recipients who develop acute cellular rejection progress to severe ductopenic rejection despite antirejection therapy requiring retransplantation.

Early acute cellular rejection usually occurs between 1 and 6 weeks post-liver transplantation and usually does not adversely affect graft or patient outcomes in patient not suffering from hepatitis C. However, late cellular rejection is associated with reduced graft survival and is usually seen with low blood levels of immunosuppressive therapy.

With current immunosuppressive drugs, signs and symptoms of acute rejection tend to be fairly mild. Most commonly, the serum bilirubin and/or transaminase

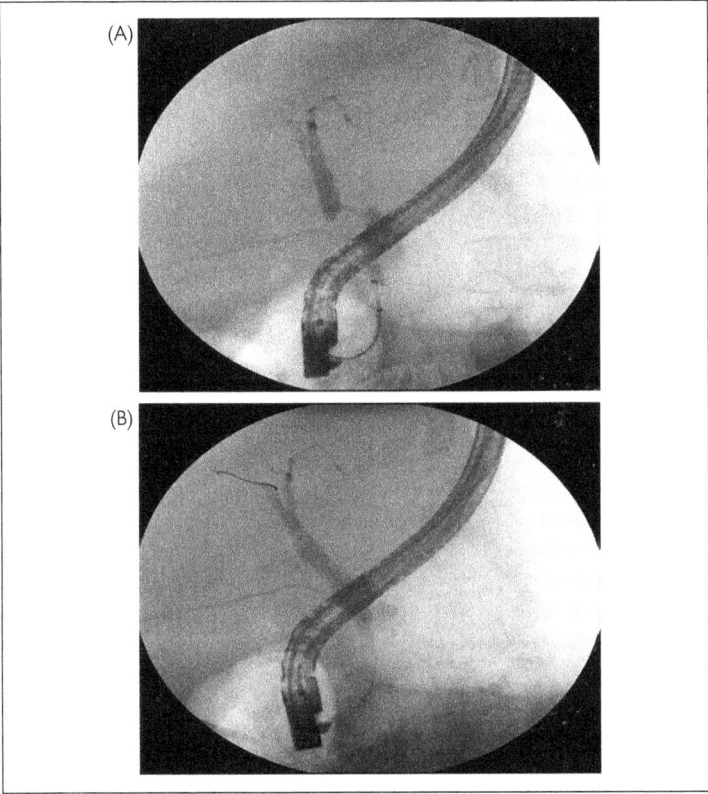

Figure 15.8. Endoscopic retrograde cholangiography images demonstrating **(A)** biliary stricture, **(B)** post-dilatation and stenting.

levels are elevated, which may be completely asymptomatic or may involve mild accompanying symptoms such as fever and malaise. The differential diagnosis must include mechanical complications (such as vascular thrombosis and bile leaks), and underlying sepsis. Ultimately, a histological assessment of the graft is required to confirm the diagnosis of acute rejection, most commonly via a percutaneous liver biopsy.

There are three major histological features associated with cellular rejection (portal inflammation, bile duct inflammation, and venular inflammation) and scored on a scale of 0 to 3. The three scores are added to arrive at a final rejection activity index (RAI). Although there is no clear-cut consensus, an RAI of 1 to 2, 3 to 4, 5 to 6, and 7 or greater is considered as borderline, mild, moderate, and severe acute rejection, respectively.

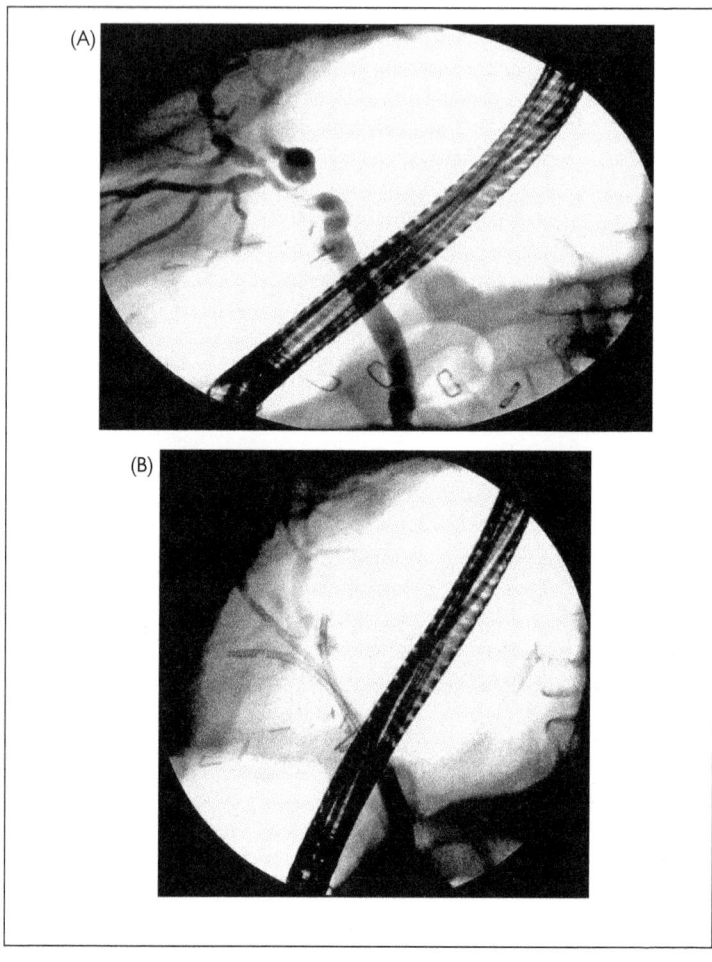

Figure 15.9. Endoscopic retrograde cholangiography images demonstrating **(A)** biliary stricture extending to three-donor duct segments and **(B)** post-stenting.

Our protocol for treatment of acute rejection depends on hepatitis C status and severity of rejection. If indeterminate or mild acute rejection—especially in a patient with hepatitis C—we treat initially by simply raising tacrolimus dose to a level around 12 to 15. If there is no response, then treat with 1000 mg of IV solumedrol for one dose (Table 15.1).

If there is moderate or severe acute rejection, then administer 1000 mg of IV solumedrol for 1 day followed by oral prednisone recycle taper (20 mg for

Table 15.1 Standard Immunosuppression—Adult Liver Transplant Program University of Pittsburgh Center

Good kidney function	Poor kidney or neurofunction	Positive cross-match	Combined liver kidney	Rejection
Prednisone or SM:	Poor kidney function defined as need for dialysis, Cr >2.5, or urine output <30cc/hr pre-op or post-op.	Prednisone or SM:	Prednisone or SM:	Solu-Medrol:
1000 mg IV before reperfusion for patients with an underlying diagnosis of auto-immune hepatitis or PSC:		1000 mg after reperfusion	1000 mg IV after reperfusion	Day #1 500 mg IV
				Day #2 250 mg IV
	Poor neurofunction is Stage 3 or 4 encephalopathy pretransplant	200 mg POD#1	20 mg starting POD#1	Day #3 125 mg IV
10 mg qdaily starting POD#1 until 12 weeks.		160 mg POD#2	Stop when FK started and therapeutic level reached	Steroid Resistant:
		120 mg POD#3		Thymoglobulin
	Prednisone or SM:	80 mg POD#4	CellCept:	1.25 mg/kg IV X 7 days
5 mg qdaily after	1000 mg IV after reperfusion	80 mg POD#5	Start immediately postop at 1.0 gm BID. Wean off over 1 month starting at 3 months posttx.	Give premeds
CellCept:	20 mg starting POD#1	40 mg POD#6		Monitor ALC
None	Stop when FK started and therapeutic level reached	20 mg for 2 weeks		
Simulect:		15 mg for 2 weeks	If unable to tolerate because of GI toxicity, may use Myfortic at 720 mg BID	
None	CellCept:	10 mg for 2 weeks		
Tacrolimus:	Start immediately postop at 1.0 gm BID. Wean off over 1 month starting at 3 months post-transplant.	7.5 mg for 2 weeks	Thymoglobulin:	
Start immediately post-op at 2.0 mg BID		5 mg for 2 weeks	1.25 mg/kg on POD#1, 3, and 5	
Adjust dose by levels		2.5 mg for 2 weeks then stop	Tacrolimus:	
0–3 months 10–12		CellCept:	Start when renal function improved	
3–6 months 8–10		Start immediately post-op at 1.0 g BID. Wean off over 1 month starting at 3 months post-transplant.		
6 months on 6–8				

(continued)

Table 15.1 (Continued)

Good kidney function	Poor kidney or neurofunction	Positive cross-match	Combined liver kidney	Rejection
	If unable to tolerate because of GI toxicity, may use Myfortic at 720 mg BID	If unable to tolerate because of GI toxicity, may use Myfortic at 720 mg BID	off dialysis, Cr <2.5, urine >30/hr) or neurological function improving at 1.0 mg BID	Give CMV & oral candida prophylaxis X 6 weeks whenever antibody therapy is given
	Simulect:	Simulect:	Adjust dose by levels	
	20 mg IV on POD#1 and POD#5	None	0–3 months 10–12	
	Or Zenapax at 1 mg/kg on POD#1 and POD#5	Tacrolimus:	3–6 months 8–10	
	Tacrolimus:	Start immediately post-op at 2.0 mg BID	6 months on 6–8	
	Start when renal function improved (off dialysis, Cr <2.5, urine >30/hr) or neurological function improving at 1.0 mg BID	Adjust dose by levels	Note: do not hold tacrolimus for >7 days.	
		0–3 months 10–12	*: For patients with underlying diagnosis of autoimmune or PSC, do not stop prednisone. Instead continue at 5 mg/day indefinitely.	
		3–6 months 8–10		
	Adjust dose by levels	6 months on 6–8		
	0–3 months 10–12	**: For patients with an underlying diagnosis of auto-immune hepatitis, do not stop prednisone. Instead once down to 5 mg/day continue indefinitely		
	3–6 months 8–10			
	6 months on 6–8			
	Note: do not hold tacrolimus for >7 days.			
	*: For patients with underlying diagnosis of auto-immune or PSC, do not stop prednisone. Instead continue at 5 mg/day indefinitely.			

ALC = Absolute Leurcocyte Count

2 weeks, 15 mg for 2 weeks, 10 mg for 2 weeks, 7.5 mg for 2 weeks, 5 mg for 2 weeks, 2.5 mg for 2 weeks, then stop). If there is no response, then we perform repeat biopsy and treat with thymoglobulin (1.25 mg/kg for 5 days) or campath (30 mg IV for one dose) if there is no improvement or worsening of biopsy findings. For treatment of chronic rejection, we increase tacrolimus level to 10 to 15 ng d/L until histological improvement is shown in a repeated liver biopsy and liver function returns to baseline. Recipients who progress to severe ductopenic chronic rejection despite antirejection therapy require retransplantation.

Selected References

Demetris, AJ, Qian, SG, Sun, H, & Fung, JJ. Liver allograft rejection: an overview of morphologic findings. *Am J Surg Pathol* 1990;14(Suppl 1):49.

Freise CE, Gillespie BW, Koffron AJ, et al. Recipient morbidity after living and deceased donor liver transplantation: findings from the A2ALL Retrospective Cohort Study. *Am J Transplant.* 2008;8(12):2569–2579.

Greif F, Bronsther OL, Van Thiel DH, et al. The incidence, timing, and management of biliary tract complications after orthotopic liver transplantation. *Ann Surg.* 1994;219(1):40–45.

Chapter 16

Kidney Transplantation

Michael C. Koprucki and Jerry McAuley

Transplant Evaluation and Contraindications

Transplantation has become the treatment of choice for patients with end-stage renal disease (ESRD), reducing mortality and increasing quality of life. The evaluation of a kidney transplant candidate involves identifying and minimizing the risks of the transplantation surgery and the required post-transplant immunosuppression, and balancing these risks with the benefits from obtaining a transplant.

Any patient with ESRD, and without absolute contraindications, should be considered for kidney transplantation. There are relatively few absolute contraindications to renal transplantation (Table 16.1). Evaluation of the potential transplant recipient should focus on identifying these contraindications early in the process. This allows the barriers to be eliminated, if possible, and also conserves the limited health-care resources involved with a full transplant evaluation. Absolute contraindications include nonadherence to therapy, drug abuse, uncontrolled psychiatric illness, active infection, malignancy, severe obesity, and uncorrectable non-kidney organ failure.

Obesity is a risk factor for poor outcomes after transplantation. However, data have not established a target weight or BMI at which transplantation should be denied, although the AST recommends a target BMI less than 30 kg/m². Obese patients may benefit from weight reduction surgery prior to transplantation. Obesity increases the risk of infections, wound complications, and mortality. Delayed graft function and long-term graft failure are more common in obese patients.

Age generally is not considered a contraindication to kidney transplantation, provided the benefit of transplantation is thought to outweigh the risks. Elderly recipients tend to have a greater number of comorbid illnesses and must be carefully evaluated to determine whether survival is expected to exceed anticipated wait times. Patients older than 60 years have improved survival after transplantation as compared to remaining on dialysis. With advances in transplant and immunosuppressive protocols resulting in better graft and patient survival, as well as a steadily increasing elderly ESRD population, a growing number of elderly patients will be referred for transplantation evaluation.

Antibodies to cytomegalovirus and Epstein-Barr virus should be tested before transplantation to guide management and prophylaxis after the transplantation. Patients should be current with their immunizations before transplantation,

Table 16.1 Contraindications to Transplantation	
1.	Non-adherence to therapy
2.	Drug abuse
3.	Uncontrolled psychiatric illness
4.	Active infection
5.	Active malignancy
6.	Severe obesity
7.	Uncorrectable non-kidney organ failure
8.	Primary oxalosis

including pneumococcal, influenza, and hepatitis B vaccines. Live vaccines should not be given in the post-transplantation setting of immunosuppression. Mycobacteria should be screened for with a thorough history of factors and possible exposure, and purified protein derivative skin testing should be performed. Transplant candidates should be screened for HIV. The recommendation is that there is poor evidence for transplantation of HIV-positive patients, although there has been recently reported success in transplantation in HIV-positive patients with CD4 T-cell counts of at least 200 cells per cubic millimeter and undetectable plasma HIV type 1 RNA levels on stable highly active antiretroviral therapy.

Patients should be screened according to the age-appropriate cancer screening guidelines for the general population. Patients with a history of malignancy who remain free of recurrence, however, should be considered for transplantation. According to the Cincinnati Transplant Tumor Registry, 54% of cases of recurrent cancer occurred when the wait time from treatment to transplantation was less than 2 years, whereas 33% occurred with wait times of 2 to 5 years, and 13% in those that waited more than 5 years. Most patients should wait 2 years after cancer treatment before transplantation, but those with breast, colon, large renal cell, and melanoma should wait at least 5 years (Table 16.2).

When evaluating a possible kidney transplant recipient, the etiology of renal failure is an important consideration because it impacts the rate of recurrence. Transplantation is still the treatment of choice because transplanted patients can experience years off dialysis. However, patients should be aware of the likelihood of recurrence of their primary renal disease before transplantation. (Table 16.3)

Recurrence of renal disease also occurs with non-glomerular disease. Primary oxalosis, in which inborn errors of hepatic glyoxylate metabolism lead to calcium oxalate deposition in the kidneys and other organs, recurs in 100% of patients without a liver transplantation to correct the underlying defect. Isolated kidney transplantation can be offered to those without severe systemic disease, whereas simultaneous kidney-liver transplantation is recommended for those with severe systemic disease.

Patients with ESRD are at risk for a number of conditions that require close monitoring and treatment in the intensive care unit (ICU). These include uremia, hyperkalemia, pericardial disease, cardiac failure, and hypertensive emergencies.

Table 16.2 Minimum Recommended Cancer-Free Waiting Period by AST Guidelines

Tumor	Recommended wait (yrs)
Renal cell cancers	None (B)
Incidental renal cancer (<5cm)	2 (B)
Symptomatic Lesions >5cm	5 (B)
Breast	5 (B)
Colon	5 (B)
Thyroid	2 (B)
Lymphoma	2 (B)
Leukemias	2 (B)
Wilm's	2 (B)
Cervix/Uterus	2 (B)
Prostate	2 (B)
Testicular	2 (B)
Bladder	2 (B)
In situ	None (B)
Melanoma	5 (B)
Basal cell skin	None (C)
Other non-melanoma skin	Unknown (C)
Myeloma	Unknown (C)

Uremia

Uremia is the clinical syndrome associated with fluid, hormonal, and electrolyte imbalances that accompany worsening renal function. Typically, uremic symptoms present clinically when estimated glomerular filtration rate (eGFR) is less than 20 mL/min/1.73 m^2. However, general symptoms such as fatigue and reduced stamina have been seen with eGFR less than 55 mL/min/1.73 m^2. With such a fundamental disruption in normal metabolism, uremia can present with a variety of symptoms, affecting every organ system. Table 16.4 lists some of the clinical features of uremia. The most common initial symptoms involve the gastrointestinal system and include anorexia, nausea, and a metallic taste to food.

Although all of the features of uremia can be seen in the ICU, the complications that often need ICU management include uremic encephalopathy, bleeding diathesis, hyperkalemia, heart failure, and pericarditis.

Uremic encephalopathy refers to the organic brain syndrome that occurs in patients with renal failure. Symptoms can vary based on both severity of renal failure and the rate at which it develops, such that symptoms are usually more

Table 16.3 Recurrence Rate and Graft Loss After Renal Transplantation

Renal disease	Recurrence rate (%)	Graft loss %
Idiopathic glomerular diseases		
FSGS	20–30	40–50
Membranous GN	10–20	50
Type I MPGN	20–30	30–40
Type II MPGN	80–100	10–20
IgA nephropathy	40–50	6–33
Anti-GBM nephritis	10	Rare
Secondary glomerular diseases		
Henoch-Schonlein purpura	15–35	10–20
Lupus nephritis	<10	Rare
HUS/TTP	28	40–50
Diabetic nephropathy	100	<5
Amyloidosis	30–40	unknown
Wegener's Granulomatosis	17	<10
Essential mixed cryoglobulinemia	50	"Frequent"
Non-glomerular disease		
Oxalosis	90–100	majority
Cystinosis	~0%	Rare
Fabry's disease	100	Rare
Sickle cell nephropathy	Rare	unknown
Scleroderma	20%	"Often"
Alport's syndrome	~0, (Anti-GBM)	~0

severe in acute kidney injury. As in other causes of metabolic encephalopathy, symptoms can vary from anorexia, lethargy, and decreased concentration in early uremia to decreased cognition in moderate uremia to asterixis, disorientation, stupor, seizures, and coma in severe uremia.

Uremic encephalopathy is an indication to initiate dialysis. Acute neurological symptoms generally reverse quickly with dialysis, although symptoms may persist for 1 to 2 days after azotemia improves. More subtle findings, as seen with progressive renal failure, may continue for longer. Also, EEG changes will persist after the patient improves clinically and may still be present several months after starting dialysis in CKD patients.

Uremic bleeding is an important complication of renal failure. Typically, uremic bleeding is cutaneous and in response to injury or procedures. Gastrointestinal bleeding is less common. Uremic bleeding is the result of impaired platelet function. Coagulation factors and the number of circulating platelets are generally normal. Platelet dysfunction in uremic patients is secondary to impaired interaction of the platelets with the vascular subendothelium, leading to impaired

Table 16.4 Clinical Features of Uremia

Neurological
Fatigue
Loss of concentration
Asterixis
Seizure
Dementia
Peripheral neuropathy
Sleep disturbances

Cardiovascular
Hypertension
Heart failure
Pericarditis
Vascular calcification
Valvular calcification

Pulmonary
Pleural effusion
Alveolar edema
Interstitial edema

Gastrointestinal
Anorexia
Nausea
Vomiting
GI hemorrhage
Delayed gastric emptying
Hiccups

Genitourinary
Amenorrhea
Erectile dysfunction

Hematologic
Platelet dysfunction
Granulocyte and lymphocyte dysfunction
Anemia

ENT
Metallic taste

Musculoskeletal
Cramps
Restless legs

Skin
Hyperpigmentation
Pruritus

Metabolic
Glucose intolerance
Hypertriglyceridemia
Hyperkalemia
Hyponatremia
Acidosis

aggregation and adhesion. The pathogenesis of uremic bleeding is not completely understood. Uremic toxins, although not the urea itself, are thought to be involved. There is no correlation between BUN and bleeding time. Also, anemia, a common complication of renal failure, hinders efficient platelet activation as more platelets circulate in the center of the blood vessel rather than near the vessel endothelial surface, as compared to when normal red blood cell numbers are present. Additionally, nitric oxide, an inhibitor of platelet aggregation, is increased in the uremic state.

For an acute correction of uremic platelet dysfunction, desmopressin (dDAVP) is the most commonly used agent. The exact mechanism of dDAVP is not known, but it is believed to act by releasing factor VIII from storage sites. The effect of dDAVP occurs within 1 hour and can last up to 24 hours. DDAVP is especially useful for uremic patients who need to undergo procedures. Also, correction of anemia will reduce bleeding time and increase platelet aggregation. Estrogen has been shown to control bleeding in uremic patients, possibly by decreasing production of L-arginine, a precursor to nitrous oxide. Estrogen decreases bleeding time with an effect in about 6 hours, with a maximum effect in 5 to 7 days, lasting for as long as 21 days. Platelet transfusion is not effective, as the platelets will acquire the functional defect from uremia. Treatment of uremic platelet dysfunction includes dialysis, although the use of anticoagulation should be minimal.

Hyperkalemia

Cardiac arrhythmias and conduction abnormalities are the most concerning clinical manifestations of hyperkalemia. Arrhythmias from hyperkalemia include sinus bradycardia, slow idioventricular rhythms, ventricular tachycardia, ventricular fibrillation, and asystole, whereas conduction abnormalities include bundle branch blocks and atrioventricular blocks. Electrocardiogram changes with hyperkalemia follow a classic pattern: peaked T waves progress to widening of the QRS complex, PR interval prolongation, QT interval shortening, decreased P wave amplitude, and, finally, a sine wave from the fusion of the QRS complex and the T wave. Clinically, EKG changes are insensitive for both the presence and the severity of hyperkalemia, and serum potassium levels must be monitored and correlated with EKG changes in each individual case. Hyperkalemia can also cause motor weakness and parasthesias, usually in an ascending pattern.

Hyperkalemia is a common medical emergency in the ICU, both as an admission diagnosis and as complication during treatment of other medical conditions. Ideally, the cause of hyperkalemia should be identified. Medication administration should be reviewed, and any offending agents, including NSAIDs, ACE inhibitors, heparin, and beta-adrenergic blockers, should be held, if possible. Also, intravenous fluids and nutritional supplementation, including tube feedings, should be reviewed to limit or eliminate potassium intake.

Regardless of the cause of hyperkalemia, the first step for treatment of severe hyperkalemia is intravenous calcium. Calcium acts to stabilize the cardiac cell membrane to protect against cardiac toxicity. The onset of action of calcium treatment is rapid, within minutes, but its duration of action is only about 30 minutes. Calcium does not lower the potassium concentration and must be followed immediately by medications that lower the potassium level. Intravenous calcium can be caustic to the surrounding tissue and is preferentially given through a central line.

After stabilization of the cell membrane, the next step in therapy involves redistributing the potassium into cells by increasing the activity of the Na-K-ATPase pump. Intravenous insulin, usually given as 10 to 20 units, has an onset of action of 30 minutes and duration of action of 2 to 3 hours. Twenty-five to 50 grams of glucose should be given over 1 hour to avoid hypoglycemia in patients receiving IV insulin. Although hypoglycemia is a risk, despite glucose administration, insulin has been shown to be effective in lowering serum potassium levels in ESRD patients. Albuterol, a beta-adrenergic agonist that increases Na-K-ATPase activity, has a similar onset and duration of action as insulin. Albuterol can be given through inhalation at a dose of 10 to 20 mg. Adverse effects include increased tachycardia and possible angina in patients with coronary artery disease. In ESRD patients, potassium reduction is addictive when both insulin and albuterol are used. Sodium bicarbonate has been used to treat hyperkalemia, based on the mechanism that if systemic pH is increased, hydrogen ions will shift out of cells and potassium will move intracellular. A number of studies have shown sodium bicarbonate to be ineffective in reducing potassium levels acutely, although there may be some benefit after several hours. Additionally, if bicarbonate is given in hypertonic solutions, such as the standard one amp of 50 meq in 50 mL, then the rise in plasma osmolality may promote water and potassium movement extracellularly. There is conflicting evidence of whether bicarbonate has additive effects on potassium lowering when administered with insulin and albuterol.

Potassium excretion is promoted by increasing distal sodium delivery and urine flow. Typically this is accomplished with intravenous furosemide and intravenous saline. In patients with anuric renal failure, this regimen will be ineffective. Resins—most notably sodium polystyrene sulfonate—are commonly used to treat hyperkalemia by binding to intestinal potassium. Although chronic use of resins can decrease potassium concentration, single-dose uses of sodium polystyrene sulfonate have been no more effective than placebo for lowering potassium levels acutely. Additionally, resins containing sorbitol have been associated with intestinal necrosis.

Dialysis is indicated for patients with ESRD or for patients whose hyperkalemia cannot be controlled with the above medical interventions. The amount of potassium removed depends on a variety of factors, the most important of which is the dialysate potassium concentration. Potassium removal can also be impacted by the total surface area of the dialyzer, the duration of dialysis, the blood flow rate, and the dialysate flow rate. Potassium levels can increase after dialysis as potassium shifts down its concentration from inside the cells to the suddenly lower potassium concentration in the extracellular space. As a result, potassium levels can be misleading immediately after dialysis and before the rebound effect.

Heart Failure

Most patients with ESRD have cardiac abnormalities. The prevalence of congestive heart failure (CHF) is 36% in patients starting dialysis. In the ICU setting, the most common complication of CHF is pulmonary edema. Although pulmonary edema in the dialysis population usually results from volume overload, ESRD patients have high rates of cardiac disease and other causes of pulmonary edema, including acute myocardial ischemia, should be investigated. Maintaining euvolemia by achieving a balance between hypervolemia and intradialytic hypotension in ICU patients on dialysis can be difficult. Hypotension in the ICU can be worsened by sepsis, hypoalbuminemia, or medications. Strategies to prevent intradialytic hypotension include avoiding rapid ultrafiltration, administering antihypertensive medications post-dialysis as opposed to pre-dialysis, and using a lower dialysis solution temperature of 35.5 to 36 degrees Celsius. Continuous renal replacement therapy provides a slower rate of volume and solute removal, allowing a relative protection against hemodynamic instability compared to conventional intermittent hemodialysis. Management of pulmonary edema in ESRD includes many therapies utilized in patients without renal failure, including oxygen therapy, vasodilators, ACE inhibitors, angiotensin II receptor blockers, and morphine.

Unique to the ESRD population, patients can develop high-output heart failure from arteriovenous fistulas (AVFs). There are numerous case reports of patients with fistulas developing worsening heart failure that improved when the fistula flow was reduced. Arteriovenous fistula high-output heart failure likely occurs more commonly in patients with underlying cardiac disease.

Pericardial Disease

Pericardial disease is common in patients with ESRD, with about 20% of patients on dialysis developing pericarditis. Pericarditis in the renal population is classified as either uremic pericarditis, which occurs in patients not dialysis or within 8 weeks of starting dialysis, or dialysis pericarditis, which occurs after 8 weeks of dialysis.

Patients with uremic pericarditis often do not have the typical EKG findings of diffuse ST elevations seen in other patients with pericarditis. The inflammatory cells of uremic exudates do not penetrate the myocardium, and it is subepicardial myocarditis that is responsible for the EKG changes. If diffuse ST elevations are present on an EKG, then another cause of pericarditis—most notably infection—must be considered. The transthoracic echocardiogram can confirm pericardial effusions in patients with ESRD. Also, ESRD patients can have an adhesive, fibrotic form of pericarditis without the presence of effusions. Dialysis pericarditis occurs primarily during periods of increased catabolism such as sepsis and trauma or during periods of inadequate dialysis from missed sessions.

For patients with uremic pericarditis, especially patients with advanced renal failure not yet on dialysis, the treatment of choice is to initiate dialysis. However, two stipulations include anticoagulation and volume removal. Given the risk of hemorrhage into the pericardial space, systemic anticoagulation should not be used. Also, fluid removal with dialysis must be done cautiously, as intravascular depletion could lead to cardiovascular collapse in patients with tamponade. For patients who develop dialysis pericarditis, intensive dialysis, usually with daily treatments, is the first line of therapy. However, response rates to intensive dialysis are significantly less, usually less than 60%, with dialysis pericarditis, as compared to uremic pericarditis, where response are typically reported as greater than 90%. Although nonsteroidal anti-inflammatory medications are used for pericarditis in non-uremic patients, they have not been shown to improve clinical outcomes in dialysis pericarditis.

With increased intensity of dialysis, the size of the effusion should be monitored. If the effusion does not resolve after 10 to 14 days, or if there is ever evidence of cardiovascular collapse, then the effusion should be drained. Generally, a pericardiotomy (where a surgical incision is made in the pericardium) is the preferred intervention. A pericardiectomy has a high success rate with rare recurrence; however, it is associated with higher morbidity, especially pulmonary complications. Increased rates of recovery with low recurrence have been associated with intrapericardial steroid instillation.

Patients with ESRD and pericarditis are at risk for cardiac tamponade. Tamponade typically manifests as dyspnea, hypotension, or mental status changes in patients with ESRD. Elevated jugular venous distention, often appreciated when tamponade occurs in non-ESRD patients, is less reliable in uremic patients because of the frequent presence of volume overload. Diagnosis should combine clinical suspicion with echocardiogram findings. Echocardiograms can show right atrial or right ventricle collapse, as intrapericardial pressure exceeds intracardiac pressure, which typically precedes clinical hemodynamic failure.

Treatment for cardiac tamponade involves rapidly decreasing the intracardiac pressure. When hemodynamically significant cardiac collapse occurs, catheter pericardiocentesis with echocardiogram guidance is the treatment of choice. Pericardiocentesis is associated with high morbidity and mortality and has a recurrence rate for hemodynamic comprise or symptomatic effusion of 70% in uremic and dialysis pericarditis. Thus, the procedure should be reserved for those with circulatory collapse. Follow-up for recurrence with an echocardiogram is recommended.

Hypertensive Emergencies

Hypertensive emergencies are defined as marked elevations in blood pressure with evidence of end-organ damage. End-organ damage from hypertensive emergencies include cerebral infarction and hemorrhage, encephalopathy, cardiac ischemia, pulmonary edema, and retinal ischemia. It is the presence of end-organ damage, and not the absolute blood pressure, that determines the urgency of treatment.

Selected Reference

Kasiske BL, Cangro CB, Hariharan S, et al. The evaluation of renal transplantation candidates: clinical practice Guidelines. *Am J Transplant* 2001;1(Suppl 2):3–95.

Chapter 17

Anesthesia Care for Kidney Transplant Recipients

Ibtesam Hilmi, Ali Abdullah, and Raymond Planinsic

Introduction

Renal transplantation (RT) provides a better quality of life and improves patient survival for up to 70% for the first 5 years when compared to 30% survival for patients on dialysis. Improvements in patient preparation, anesthetic care, and surgical technique make RT a relatively safe procedure and favorably impact the organ and patient outcome. The relatively long cold ischemia time that kidney allograft can tolerate when compared to other solid organs allows adequate time for recipient preparation. Most of the time the recipients arrive to the operating room well-prepared, dialyzed, volume-optimized, and sometimes with immune suppressive regimen started.

Pre-Operative Preparation

Patient and graft outcome are significantly improved if RT is performed before patient requires dialysis. If patients have already commenced dialysis, then the shorter period of time the patient has been on dialysis, the better the outcome. Patients with end-stage renal disease (ESRD) usually present with multiple medical problems that may or may not be related to renal failure or to the therapeutic interventions.

Pre-Operative Testing

Exercise tolerance test is currently recommended for patients with ESRD who have diabetes mellitus, and for those older than age 50 years, this test has low specificity and sensitivity and may not predict the peri-operative cardiac risks. Myocardium perfusion scan has better sensitivity and specificity and should be considered in these cases. Adenosine or dobutamine stress ECHO are the most commonly used screening tests, are less invasive, and offer the ability to evaluate the myocardial performance and valve functions and detect the possibility of pulmonary hypertension.

Screening tests for viral hepatitis (especially HCV), which is fairly common in patients on hemodialysis, should be performed. The high incidence of HCV results from contaminated equipment or blood transfusions. However, chronic infection with HCV by itself may lead to glomerulonephritis-induced ESRD. Other commonly performed tests are Hb/Hct, coagulation tests, arterial blood gas, and electrolytes. Dialysis will correct some of these problems, but it can create problems of its own. Timing of dialysis is essential, and such timing is most often possible in elective RT from a live donor. Patients receiving cadaveric RT may arrive to the operating room immediately after dialysis or if they have missed their scheduled dialysis. The care providers have to be prepared for any problem that results from such circumstances.

Intra-Operative Monitoring

Monitoring is crucial for intra-operative management of patients with ESRD who are undergoing RT. The intra-operative monitoring may be extended to the post-operative phase to manage fluid and medication administration. The choice of monitoring should be tailored to the individual patient and the presence or absence of comorbidities. Factors that are of importance in the choice of monitoring include surgical technique, the experience of the surgical team, possibility of blood loss, the experience of the anesthesiologist in certain monitoring techniques or equipment, and the availability of monitoring technology.

Securing an arterial catheter is essential for continuous blood pressure monitoring and blood sampling for arterial blood gas and other testing. Although it is very desirable to secure an arterial access, it is not always possible to find a viable peripheral artery to canulate. Availability of Doppler ultrasound may help in establishing arterial access.

Central venous pressure (CVP) monitoring is widely used during RT surgery; the accuracy of CVP to monitor left ventricle pre-load status is still debatable.

Transesophageal echocardiography is an excellent tool to monitor the pre-load as well as other hemodynamic and cardiac parameters, but it is very much operator-dependent and requires extensive training.

Pulmonary artery catheter (PAC) has the same limitations of the CVP but remains the gold standard for measuring the pulmonary artery pressure. The addition of continuous monitoring of cardiac output (CO), right ventricular end-diastolic volume, right ventricular ejection fraction, and SVO_2 to the PAC improved the quality of data that PAC can provide.

New technologies in clinical practice include noninvasive cardiovascular monitoring utilizing the arterial tracing to calculate beat-to-beat CO, cardiac index, stroke volume variation, stroke volume index, and pulse pressure variation. This technology may be helpful, especially in patients with difficult central venous access resulting from thrombosed or stenosed veins from multiple previous venous cannulation, which is seen frequently in these patients.

Promising new technology utilizes the principle of bioreactance, which analyzes beat-by-beat changes in the intrathoracic fluid content on transmission of electoral signals through the thorax and relates these changes to the absolute value of SV, calculating CO and other hemodynamic parameters. Although these monitors have been available for several years, there are no studies to validate their usefulness in RT recipients.

Pharmacokinetics and Pharmacodynamics of End-Stage Renal Disease

End-stage renal disease affects all drugs excreted by the kidneys. In addition, it may modify disposition of drugs through changes in plasma protein binding, volume of distribution, and hepatic clearance by enzyme induction or inhibition.

Lipophilic drugs such as benzodiazepine and barbiturate have shown an increase in volume of distribution accompanied by increased clearance. The increase in the availability of the free portion of the lipophilic drugs will result in unchanged rate of elimination. The pharmacokinetics and pharmacodynamic of propofol and etomidate are very much unchanged and can be used safely in patients with ESRD.

Opioids

The pharmacokinetics and pharmacodynamics of the most commonly used opioids (fantanly, alfantentanil, sufentanil, and remifentanil) are not changed by ESRD and can be used safely without dose adjustment. Meperidine metabolism produces an active metabolite (normeperidine). This is normally excreted by the kidney and can accumulate to produce neurotoxicity in patients with ESRD. Morphine metabolism yields active metabolites (morphine-6-β glucuranide [M6G] and morphine-3-β glucuranide [M3G]), which are normally excreted by the kidney. M6G and M3G accumulate in patients with ESRD and slowly cross the blood–brain barrier, leading to serious respiratory depression. Morphine and meperidine can cause histamine release that may destabilize the delicate hemodynamic balance in patients with ESRD. It is preferable not to use these narcotics in this patient population. Hydromorphone is safely used in patients with ESRD—especially for post-operative pain control. However, whichever opioid is used, close monitoring is the key to prevent unwanted side effects.

Muscle Relaxants

Succinylcholine is a depolarizing muscle relaxant that may be safely used in patients with ESRD if the serum K^+ is normalized by dialysis or other means of renal supportive therapy. Succinylcholine increases serum K+ by 0.5 to 1.0 mEq/L that may last up to 15 minutes. Serum K+ of less than 5.5 mEq/L should be aimed before using succinylcholine to facilitate endotracheal intubation.

Depolarizing muscle relaxant is preferable in patients who are at high risk of pulmonary aspiration as in ESRD resulting from autonomic gastropathy, obesity, or on peritoneal dialysis with significant volume of dialysate fluid left in. Most of the modern non-depolarizing muscle relaxants can be used in ESRD, such as rocuronium and vacuronium, with some prolongation of action to be expected. Cisatracurium is metabolized by ester hydrolysis and Hofmann degradation, which is completely independent of renal or hepatic function. Cisatracurium may be considered as a drug of choice in patients with liver or renal failure; however, histamine release can occur with its use but is usually harmless. Pancronium is a long-acting muscle relaxant, which has active metabolites cleared by the kidney with 30% of the parent drug. Reversal of neuromuscular blockade with glucopyrolate and neostigmine can be safely carried out in patients with ESRD. Neostigmine may show slight prolongation of action, an effect that could be desirable in these patients because of prolongation of action of most of the neuromuscular blockers.

Inhalational Anesthetics

The issue of inorganic fluoride and its nephrotoxicity has been well established with methoxyflurane, which is no longer in use. Sevoflurane, which is one of the new generation of inhalational agents, is minimally metabolized in the liver to yield hexa-fluoro-isopropanol and inorganic fluoride. The serum levels of inorganic fluoride after sevoflurane use can reach a higher level than enflurane when used in same MAC/hour. However, it is still below the toxic level (50 µMol/L). Sevoflurane degrades to compound-A by carbon dioxide absorbers containing barium hydroxide lime or soda lime when used at a low flow (<1.5 L/minute). The heat and humidity generated in the gas mixture is capable of inducing this degradation of sevoflurane in the anesthetic breathing circuit. Compound-A has been shown to be nephrotoxic in animals. Although the safety of sevoflurane in patients with renal dysfunction is still not clear, its use during RT has not received much attention and not much is known about its effects on the renal allograft. Neither desflurane nor isoflurane increases the serum levels of inorganic fluoride, and they have no known nephrotoxic effects and can be used safely in patients with ESRD undergoing RT. In general, the indirect effects of anesthetic agents and techniques with added factors of surgical trauma and stress have more pronounced effects on the renal functions than the direct effects. The indirect effects of anesthesia and surgical stress on the autonomic nervous system, the cardiovascular system, and the humoral modulation can dramatically influence renal functions. Whether such factors can influence the recipient and renal allograft outcome requires further studies. Overall, the direct effects of most, if not all, anesthetic medications on the renal functions and renal welfare are quite benign.

Positive Inotropic Medications

Vasopressor or positive inotropic agents may be needed during RT surgery to increase CO and renal perfusion pressure. Pressors may be helpful in some patients to balance the CVS effects of anesthetic agents or to rescue hemo-dynamic stability during graft re-perfusion. Although dopamine is the most commonly used agent during RT, there is little evidence to support its use in improving renal perfusion and/or renal graft performance. Dopamine may induce tachycardia and arrhythmia, which may compromise myocardial perfu-sion and adversely affect patient outcome. Recently, some studies have shown fenoldopam (an agent with selective dopamine-1 receptor agonist) to improve renal perfusion. However, fenoldopam is not without side effects; tachycardia and systemic hypotension may occur. Powerful α-agonist agents such as norepi-nephrine, which increases perfusion pressure, may have effects on renal blood flow; these effects have not been fully studied. Vasopressin, another agent with strong vasoconstriction effects on multiple vascular beds, may decrease the blood flow to the splanchnic area and may compromise renal blood flow.

Whenever a vasopressor agent is required to improve cardiac performance and/or increase renal perfusion pressure, several things should be considered: the presence of cardiovascular diseases, the pre-load status of the recipients, and the effects of the anesthetic agents or technique or the CVS.

Post-Operative Care

When considering the type of post-operative care of RT recipients, multiple fac-tors require careful consideration by the anesthesiologist. These include:

1. The presence of the comorbidity, such as cardiovascular diseases, obstruc-tive sleep apnea, compromised respiratory function, obesity, and age.
2. Intra-operative course and complications, such as massive bleeding, requirement for continuous inotropic support, and anesthesia-related complications (aspiration, unexpected medication side effects).
3. Renal allograft performance. Resumption of renal function is a very impor-tant factor in determination of the type of post-operative care these patients will require. Primary graft failure or delayed graft function may simply mean that the recipient is in urgent need of HD to optimize pre-load status and correct any acid-base and electrolytes disturbances.

Intensive care setting is an appropriate option for RT recipients when any of the aforementioned scenarios occurs.

Selected Reference

Lemmens, Harry JM. Kidney transplantation: recent developments and recommendations for anesthetic management. *Anesthesiology Clin N Am* 2004;(22):651–662.

Chapter 18

Kidney Transplantation-Surgical Techniques

Abhideep Chaudhary, Ron Shapiro, and Martin Wijkstrom

Küss first described the iliac fossa technique of kidney transplantation in 1951, and since then the surgical technique has changed very little (Shapiro, 1998).

Preparation of the Patient

Kidney transplant is considered clean-contaminated surgery, so prophylactic antibiotics are administered 30 minutes before skin incision. A first generation cephalosporin (e.g., cefazolin) is routinely used, but if the patient is allergic to penicillin, a combination of vancomycin and ciprofloxacin can be considered. Many surgeons prefer to distend the bladder with normal saline (may be supplemented with antibiotics 0.25% Neomycin GU irrigant or 1 g cephazolin in 1 L of saline) while clamping the Foley.

Exposure

Kidney transplantation is a heterotopic procedure, with the kidney placed in iliac fossa in an extraperitoneal location, which allows for easy access for percutaneous renal biopsy. The right iliac fossa is usually preferred because of the more superficial location of the iliac vein on this side; however, left iliac fossa should be used if the recipient may be a candidate for future pancreas transplant, if it is a second transplant, or if there is significant arterial disease on the right side. In children (<15 kg body weight) where the iliac vessels are small or in adults with previous renal transplants, the kidney is placed intra-abdominally, with vessels anastomosed to common iliac vessels or directly to the aorta and vena cava.

Preparation of the Kidney

A varying degree of dissection of the kidney is required, particularly with a deceased donor kidney before the kidney can be transplanted. The preparation of the deceased donor kidney usually is performed before the start of transplant procedure to assure that the organ is transplantable.

The deceased donor kidney usually comes with a segment of aorta and inferior vena cava, which are trimmed according to size of vessels and recipient body habitus. At the donor procurement operation, it is important is to keep the donor renal artery or arteries in continuity with a patch of donor aorta (Carrel patch), making the end-to-side anastomosis easier and facilitating the anastomosis of multiple renal arteries.

With a kidney from a living donor, the donor artery and vein are shorter than with a deceased donor kidney, as the donor vena cava and aorta are not available. In the case of multiple arteries, reconstruction usually is done on the back table, and either the arteries are joined together at their orifices to form a common trunk (V-plasty) or a smaller artery is anastomosed end-to-side to a larger renal artery. It is important to have the lower polar artery revascularized because this can occasionally give rise to the ureteric blood supply.

Vascular Anastomosis and Reperfusion

The renal vein is anastomosed first, end-to-side to the external iliac vein, and the renal artery is anastomosed end-to-side to the external iliac artery. The kidney can be kept cold during the implantation either by wrapping the kidney in an ice blanket or by topical irrigation with cold saline. Furosemide (1 mg/kg) and mannitol (1 g/kg) are infused slowly as the vessels are anastomosed. Before the release of the vascular clamps, a dose of 500 mg methylprednisolone is given. Following reperfusion, care is taken to assure adequate hemostasis, and another dose of furosemide is given.

Ureteral Reconstruction

The important principle is to attach the ureter to the bladder mucosa in a tension-free manner and to cover the distal 1 cm of ureter with a submucosal tunnel, thus protecting against reflux. Foley catheter drainage of the bladder is required for about 3 days, unless there are bladder abnormalities that may necessitate drainage for up to 7 days. Whatever technique is used for the ureteral anastomosis, an indwelling stent may be placed at the discretion of the transplant surgeon. Routine stenting may not be necessary for patients at low risk for urologic complications. If a stent is placed, then it should be removed 6 weeks after transplantation.

Immunosuppression

The success of modern transplantation is in large part related to the successful development of effective immunosuppressive agents. The most important goal of immunosuppression is avoidance of acute rejection, as even a single episode of acute rejection may predispose to chronic changes and may reduce long-term graft survival. Immunosuppressive agents used for kidney transplant patients can be categorized according to their use:

1. Induction agents—those used for a limited interval at the time of transplant
2. Maintenance agents—those used long term for maintenance of immunosuppression
3. Anti-rejection drugs—those used for a short time or in high doses to reverse an acute rejection episode

Induction Therapy

All recipients require immunosuppressive therapy at the time of transplantation. The goal of induction immunosuppression is to provide powerful immunosuppression peri-transplant, decrease the overall incidence of rejection, and permit (if desired) delay in introducing other maintenance agents such as calcineurin inhibitors.

Agents used for induction therapy are classified as polyclonal (e.g., anti-thymocyte globulin: Thymoglobulin®) or monoclonal antibodies (e.g., basiliximab: anti-interleukin (IL)-2 receptor inhibitory antibody, Simulect®; or alemtuzumab: depleting anti-CD52 antibody; Campath®).

An important issue is which agent should be used. Anti-thymocyte globulin and alemtuzumab are more potent induction agents but are associated with side effects that can include fever, leukopenia, thrombocytopenia, and an increased risk of CMV and and other infections, whereas IL-2 receptor antagonist use is associated with fewer side effects but less potency. With this view, more aggressive immunosuppression is justified in patients who are at significantly increased risk of rejection. Clinical practice guidelines from Kidney Disease Improving Global Outcomes relating to the care of the kidney transplant patient were published in 2009. As per these guidelines, all patients should get induction treatment and suggest the use of lymphocyte-depleting agents, which are potent immunosuppressive agents, for patients at higher risk for acute rejection. Recipients are considered to be at high immunological risk for acute rejection if one or more of the following is present:

- Increased number of human leukocyte antigen (HLA) mismatches
- Younger recipient and older donor age
- African-American ethnicity (in the United States)
- Panel reactive antibody (PRA) greater than 0%
- Presence of a donor-specific antibody
- Blood group incompatibility
- Delayed onset of graft function
- Cold ischemia time greater than 24 hours

At UPMC, we utilize induction therapy for all patients undergoing kidney transplantation. The choice of agent depends on hepatitis C status and history of malignancy. For the majority of patients who are hepatitis C negative, a single infusion of alemtuzumab (30 mg) is given after premedication with 10 to 15 mg/kg methylprednisolone or in the operating room after induction of anesthesia with a second dose of methylprednisolone repeated before graft reperfusion. For patients who are hepatitis C-positive, two doses of basiliximab (20 mg per dose) are given: the first dose in the operating room after induction of anesthesia, and the second dose on post-operative days 2 through 4. Alternatively, in hepatitis C-positive patients at increased risk for rejection, 1 mg/kg anti-thymocyte globulin in the operating room and daily for the first 4 days after transplantation is a reasonable alternative.

Maintenance Immunosuppression

Maintenance immunosuppressive medication is life-long treatment to prevent acute rejection and deterioration of graft function. From just two drugs available in the 1960s, azathioprine and prednisone, the therapeutic armamentarium for transplant patients has broadened significantly, with a variety of drug combinations and protocols available currently. At most centers, calcineurin inhibitors form the basis of immunosuppressive protocols. These drugs have been used as monotherapy and/or in combination with an antimetabolite and/or steroid. Induction with alemtuzumab followed by tacrolimus monotherapy has been successfully used in kidney transplantation with low acute rejection rates. It is important to note that for all protocols, monitoring drug levels and maintaining calcineurin inhibitor levels within a specified drug range seem critical to prevent acute rejection episodes early post-transplant. Prospective randomized trials have shown a lower incidence of acute rejection when mycophenolate is added to calcineurin inhibitor-based protocols.

Calcineurin inhibitor-free protocols have been devised. The major goal of such protocols is to avoid the nephrotoxicity associated with use of calcineurin inhibitors. The combination of sirolimus and mycophenolate has been used to achieve these results. Although nephrotoxicity can be avoided, relatively high doses of both drugs need to be used, rejection rates are high, and patient and graft survival rates are inferior.

Historically, the principal theme of maintenance immunosuppression has been to use higher doses of immunosuppression early post-transplantation when the risk of acute rejection is highest, and then to reduce doses as the risk of acute rejection diminishes over time.

Current maintenance immunosuppression for kidney transplantation at most centers includes calcineurin-inhibitor-based triple-drug therapy (mostly tacrolimus/mycophenolate mofetil/steroids). Locally, we use double immunosuppressive therapy with tacrolimus and mycophenolate mofetil.

Tacrolimus is started on post-operative day 1 and given twice daily for the first 6 months, with 12-hour trough level targets of 8 to 10 ng/mL and target trough levels 5 to 7 ng/mL thereafter. Mycophenolate mofetil is also started on post-operative day 1 at 500 mg twice daily. Dose reductions may be needed secondary to neutropenia or gastrointestinal side effects. Steroids are avoided routinely.

Immune Monitoring

Immunological monitoring remains an area of active clinical investigation. At UPMC, we perform enzyme-linked immunosorbent assays (ELISAs) to screen for the presence of Class I and II anti-HLA IgG antibodies pre-transplant and every 3 months post-transplant. The results provide insight into the state of humoral immune reactivity. We perform Luminex bead flow-cytometry to identify donor-specific antibody (DSA) in recipient serum if the ELISA class I or II antibodies are 10% or greater, or when antibody-mediated rejection (AMR) is suspected. As additional useful immunological monitoring markers become available, they will be adopted to the panel of serial testing.

Prophylactic Antimicrobial Treatment (See Chapter 9)

Immunosuppressed kidney transplant recipients are at risk for developing infections. The occurrence of certain types of infections as well as the organisms involved tends to follow a general temporal pattern in the post-transplant period.

Infections are the leading cause of morbidity and mortality in the early post-transplant period. Peri-operative surgical antibiotic prophylaxis with broad spectrum antibiotics are used for prevention of wound infections. In addition, aggressive pulmonary physiotherapy and early ambulation reduces the incidence of hospital-acquired pneumonia.

In the 1- to 6-month post-transplant period, kidney transplant recipients are predisposed to infections characteristic of those in patients with T-cell deficiency. Cytomegalovirus (CMV) infection is most common in this period and should be considered in any recipient presenting with fever, arthralgia, myalgia, or other vague symptoms. Acute rejection and recipient age are independent risk factors for CMV infection, and episodes of rejection and serological status of the donor and the recipient are independent risk factors for CMV disease (the highest risk is with a CMV-seropositive donor to a CMV-seronegative recipient). The use of depleting antibodies for the treatment of rejection also predisposes to CMV infection. Because of the frequency and severity of disease, a considerable effort should be made to prevent and treat CMV infection in renal transplant recipients.

We use oral valganciclovir for a period of 6 months for all recipients. We also perform CMV polymerase chain reaction (PCR) on all recipients every month for 6 months and then every 3 months for 2 years post-transplant.

Epstein-Barr virus (EBV) can be serious and may present as lymphoproliferative disease. The incidence of EBV disease is higher among patients who acquire EBV infection from the donor and those who get depleting antibody induction before transplant. So for EBV-negative recipients who get a kidney from EBV-positive donors, we use 100 mg/kg cytogam intravenously on post-operative day 1 and continue valganciclovir (dose-adjusted based on kidney function) for 1 year, in addition to monitoring EBV by performing quantitative EBV PCR testing monthly for the first 12 months and then every other month for the subsequent year.

Other opportunistic infections commonly seen in the 1- to 6-month post-transplant period include *Pneumocystis carinii*, *Listeria*, herpes, and fungal. We start prophylactic antimicrobials in the immediate post-operative period. All patients receive trimethoprim-sulfamethoxazole (Bactrim®) daily for 3 months, followed by three times a week for the duration of immunosuppression. Bactrim is not only effective for prophylaxis of *Pneumocystic carinii*, *Listeria*, and nocardia infections but also helps minimize the incidence of urinary tract infection post-transplant. We also administer nystatin to all recipients for 4 months post-transplant for prophylaxis of oral candidiasis.

BK virus infection is only seen in immunosuppressed patients. High titers of BK virus detected by PCR in urine and blood are predictive of development of graft BK nephropathy. We perform screening for polyoma/BK virus in plasma and the urine. Urine and plasma PCR is performed monthly for the first 6 months and then every 3 months for the first 2 years. In all allograft biopsies, staining for BK viral inclusions is routine and *in situ* hybridization for BK/polyoma virus is performed. Reduction of immunosuppression is critical and can reduce rates of graft loss to BK virus nephropathy significantly. We consider viremia greater than 10^4 copies/mL blood, or evidence of BK-associated nephropathy on biopsy (*in situ* hybridization) to be significant and indication to treat. Immunosuppression is reduced by adjusting tacrolimus trough levels to 5 to 6 ng/mL, or lower, and discontinuing mycophenolate mofetil or sirolimus as applicable. We use low-dose intravenous cidofovir treatment rarely for viremia but always for BK nephropathy. We consider the use leflunomide in cases not well controlled with cidofovir.

Beyond 6 months post-transplant, the infectious profile of patients with stable graft function is usually similar to that of the general population. However, a few patients may have complications from viral infections like EBV-associated lymphoproliferative disease, CMV reactivation leading to CMV retinitis, or other invasive disease (pulmonary, hepatic, and gastrointestinal). Patients who are on higher doses of immunosuppression because of rejection or who receive long-term steroids are at risk for a similar spectrum of opportunistic infections seen in the 1- to 6-month post-transplant period.

UPMC Immune Suppression Protocol for Kidney and Pancreas Transplant

Living donor kidney recipients	Deceased donor kidney recipients	Sensitized kidney patients receiving either plasma pheresis/IVIG or IVIG/rituximab	Pancreas transplantation	HCV+ kidney recipients
Methylprednisolone: After induction of anesthesia, 500 mg IV (adjusted for smaller pediatric recipients) ×2. Benadryl, Tylenol, & Pepcid, one dose prior to Alemtuzumab and one dose during the arterial anastomosis **Alemtuzumab:** • Adults: 30 mg • Pediatric: 0.4–0.5 mg/kg (pts <60kg) • given intra-operatively after induction of anesthesia over 2–3 hours, prior to cross-clamp release **Tacrolimus:** Post-operative day 1 3 mg post-operative bid (adjusted for pediatric patients), with target level of 8.5–10 mg/mL for the first 4 months following transplantation; 4 month to 1 year 5–7 mg/mL. **Mycophenolate:** Post-operative day 1, 500 mg post-operative bid mycophenolate mofetil or 360 mg mycophenolate sodium (Myfortic)—for all patients except HLA-identical living related donor recipients	Same regimen	**Tacrolimus / MMF:** Started on 1st day of plasma pheresis/IVIG aiming for a target Tacrolimus level of 10mg/mL, MMF 500 mg bid, Continued post-transplantation **Methylprednisolone and Alemtuzumab:** As per living donor and deceased donor regimen	**Campath:** Given as for living and deceased donor kidneys **Tacrolimus/MMF:** Started post-operatively on post-operative day 1 aiming for a target Tacrolimus level of 10 ng/mL, MMF 500–1000 mg po bid Pancreas after kidney • <3 months: Basiliximab 20 mg on day 0, 4 • 3–6 months: Campath 1H 20 mg • 6 months: Campath 1H 30 mg	**IL-2 receptor antagonists** Basiliximab 20 mg day in OR and post-operative day 4 For deceased donor recipients with long (>24 hours) CIT, or high PRA, consider thymoglobulin 1 mg/kg in the OR and for the first 4 days post-operatively Tacrolimus post-operative day 1, target level 12 mg/mL MMF 1 gram bid or Myfortic 720 mg bid

Acute cellular rejection Banff 1A-1B	Banff 2A/steroid-resistant rejection	Humoral rejection (C4d-positive, DSA+)	CNI toxicity	BKV	Neutropenia
• Solumedrol 500 mg IV qd x3 (or 10 mg/kg in pediatric patients) • Adjustment of tacrolimus and MMF dosing • Borderline— Some variability, ranging from 1 to 3 doses of steroids and adjustment of tacrolimus and mmf dosing	• IVIG 500 mg/kg/d x4 or • Thymoglobulin 1mg/kg/d x 7–10 d or • Campath 1H 30 mg IV	• Plasmapheresis/IVIG 100 mg/kg 3x/wk; consider Rituximab, Bortezomib if not effective • Can also administer a few boluses of steroids at the discretion of the treating clinician if there is a component of acute cellular rejection	• Reduce CNI dose • Consider conversion to Sirolimus	• Viremia 10⁴, nephropathy • Reduce tacrolimus dosing. Aim for level of 5–6 ng/mL or lower • If on MMF or Sirolimus, reduce by 50% • Consider Cidofovir 0.25–0.33 mg/kg/wk for nephropathy • Consider leflunomide 100mg/d x 5d; then 40–60 mg/d post-operatively (target levels 50–100)	Defined as ANC <500 Neupogen—300 µg sc qd x 3; alternatively, 480 µg sc x1 May need to repeat as needed If refractory, may need to reduce valganciclovir dose to 450 mg qod or even discontinue it; alternatively, may need to reduce MMF dose to 250 mg bid (or Myfortic 180 mg bid); alternatively, consider reducing Bactrim to M, W, F (this would be less likely)

Immunological monitoring	Infection prophylaxis	Infectious disease monitoring	De novo DSA (in previously transplanted patients)	Anti-coagulation

• Class I and II ELISA at 1 and 3 months, 1 and 3 months after any major change, and every 3 months chronically
 	
• Cylex studies performed at the same time points
	• Nystatin 5 mL swish and swallow four times daily for 4 months
	• Valganciclovir 450 mg once daily post-operatively for 6 months (can reduce to 3 months in CMV-seropositive patients or CMV—to—cases), bactrim single strength one tablet daily for 3 months, then M, W, F
	• For EBV+ donors / EBV- recipients
	  ○ Cytogam 100 mg/kg IV on post-operative day 1
	  ○ Valganrciclovir 450 mg/d (or pediatric equivalent) x 1 year
	  ○ Monthly EBV PCRs x 1 year, then q 2–3 months
	• For patients with bactrim allergy, Dapsone 100 mg/d, or inhalational pentamidine 300 mg/month, or mepron 1500 mg/d
		BK Virus:
		Urine and plasma PCR monthly for the first 6 months, and then every 3 months for the first 2 years
		CMV:
		PCR monthly for the first 6 months, and then every 3 months x 2 years
			Stable creatinine: Abandon spaced weaning (if on spaced weaning) to once daily tacrolimus.
			Increase tacrolimus to bid from qd if on qd.
			Consider MMF
			Rising creatinine:
			Biopsy, treat as for humoral rejection
				Routine kidney:
				ASA 81 mg/d x 3 mo → indefinitely
				Pancreas:
				ASA 81 mg/d plus enoxaparin 0.5 mg/kg/d (for SPK), 1 mg/kg/d (for PAK, PTA) x 1 week or until discharge
				At risk: ASA 81 mg/d, enoxaparin 0.5 mg/kg/d, (re)start coumadin at 1 week

Fluid Management and Renal Replacement Therapy

The goal of fluid management is to achieve adequate cardiac filling pressures for optimal cardiac output. Patients with known significant cardiac diastolic or systolic dysfunction or other significant medical comorbidity may be monitored by central venous pressures or pulmonary artery catheter to maintain central venous pressure at 8 to 12 mmHg, or pulmonary capillary wedge pressures at 8 to 10 mmHg. There has been an increasing interest in using minimally invasive monitoring devices that measure cardiac output, PPV and SVV, which are more sensitive and specific in determining preload responsiveness.

In the standard case, regardless of whether the patient is on dialysis, we usually give 2 to 4 L of crystalloids in the operating room before the vascular anastomosis is completed. Typically, if the patient is already on dialysis, then he arrives to the operating room in a hypovolemic state. At the time of venous anastomosis, we give intravenous diuretics; 1 g/kg body weight of mannitol and 1 mg/kg body weight furosemide to encourage the new kidney to start diuresing.

The main risk for the hypovolemic patient is hypotension and graft thrombosis. Hypervolemia may lead to hypertension, pulmonary edema, and increased oxygen requirement, leading to difficulty with extubating the patient, and may necessitate an otherwise unnecessary ICU admission. Other clinical parameters that can be used in the assessment of volemic state include plain chest radiograph to evaluate for pulmonary edema, thirst in the awake patient, and the degree of moistness of oral mucus membranes.

Patients who are monitored in the ICU post-transplant most likely will have invasive monitoring. In such cases, fluid management can be based on direct venous filling pressures. Most kidney recipients, however, are able to go to the floor after discharge from the post-operative care unit. Fluid management in those patients is based on a routine protocol that can be individualized (e.g., in patients where the new kidney is anuric). Our fluid protocol is based on urine output: for urine output less than 300 mL/hour, we replace with equal amount of fluids; for urine output greater than 300 mL/hour, we replace 80% of the output.

The choice of intravenous fluid depends on the patient's need, usually half-normal saline in diabetic patients, and half-normal saline supplemented with 50 mEq of sodium bicarbonate and 25 g dextrose per liter in non-diabetic patients. As a rule, diabetic patients are on an insulin infusion peri-operatively, to control blood sugars tightly. Both surgical stress as well as the use of peri-operative corticosteroids (used for both prophylaxis against potential cytokine storm post-alemtuzumab infusion and for immunosuppression) may cause hyperglycemia.

Post-Transplant Dialysis

For patients receiving a kidney transplant before needing renal replacement therapy (pre-emptive transplantation), post-transplant dialysis is rarely needed. For patients already receiving routine hemodialysis or peritoneal dialysis, the need to perform dialysis within a week of the transplant is defined as delayed graft function (DGF). Indications for dialysis are the same as for dialysis pre-transplant and include hyperkalemia or other electrolyte imbalance, fluid overload (pulmonary edema), metabolic acidosis, or pericarditis. The risk of DGF is mostly related to the quality of the donor organ; risk factors are brain death of the organ donor, inotropic support of the donor, donor creatinine, cold ischemia time, age, comorbidities of the donor, and so forth. A large analysis of kidney transplant recipients in the United States showed that the incidence of DGF is 42% in recipients of kidneys from donation after cardiac death donors and 23% in recipients of brain-dead donors. Of 1200 recipients of living donor kidneys at one institution, only 1.5% experienced DGF; national data suggest an incidence of 5% to 6% in living donor recipients. Primary nonfunction occurs less frequently.

Delayed graft function, a term sometimes used interchangeably with acute tubular necrosis, is an independent risk factor for poor long-term graft function and survival. The exact mechanisms responsible for DGF and downstream events are not clearly delineated but are related to ischemia-reperfusion injury. Acute injury to the transplanted kidney predisposes to acute rejection and to chronic graft nephropathy.

Blood Pressure Management

The goal peri-operative systolic blood pressure is 130 to 140 mmHg, or mean arterial pressure 70 to 90 mmHg. The surgical risk of untreated hypertension is primarily bleeding. Most patients are treated for hypertension pre-operatively. We ask our living donor kidney recipients to not take their home anti-hypertensive regimen the morning of the transplant. The same is requested of our diseased donor kidney recipients, but the possibility to interrupt scheduled medication may be limited by the time the patient is called to the hospital for transplant.

Post-transplantation, it is important to resume pre-transplant anti-hypertensive medications—particularly beta-blockade and clonidine—to prevent rebound hypertension. Early post-operation hypertension is typically treated as in any monitored patient. In the immediate post-operative period, hypertension can be attributed to pain, hypothermia, and hypoxia. After these possibilities have been excluded, first-line therapy consists of single doses of intravenous short-acting beta-blockers (labetolol, metoprolol), followed by intravenous hydralazine, or intravenous ACE-inhibitor (enalapril). If continuous infusion of anti-hypertensive medication is required, then the calcium-channel blocker nicardipine is a good first-line agent, closely followed by esmolol (as tolerated by the heart rate).

Hypotension in a post-transplant patient is worrisome, and the first step should be to identify the cause. Hypotension most commonly is related to bleeding, acute myocardial infarction, or hypovolemia. Less commonly, hypotension may be secondary to electrolyte disturbance, sympathetic blockade (i.e., initiation of spinal or epidural analgesia), drug induced (from intra-operative use of beta-blockade), or anaphylactic reaction to a new medication. The appropriate investigations need to be initiated but should not delay treatment. Invasive monitoring should be considered, and if appropriate response is not achieved after fluid resuscitation, then vasopressors and or inotropes should be started. Dopamine, norepinephrine, or vasopressin are all reasonable agents.

Post-Operative Complications

Wound Complications

Both infectious and noninfectious wound complications are similar to those seen in general surgical patients. The incidence of superficial wound infections and for dehiscence and incisional hernias is 2% to 5%. Li et al. (2005) at the University of Maryland reported on 2499 kidney transplant recipients, of whom 41 (1.6%) developed an incisional hernia that required plastic surgery-assisted repair. Most lower quadrant defects were repaired with tensor fascia lata grafts and most midline defects with a component separation technique.

Bleeding

Post-transplant bleeding is a relatively uncommon complication of transplant surgery. Factors contributing to increased risk of post-transplant bleeding include pre-transplant hemodialysis, the use of anticoagulation medications (aspirin, Coumadin, clopidogrel, etc.), pre- and peri-operative plasmapheresis, multiple renal arteries necessitating vascular reconstruction, and post-operative hypertension.

Hemodialysis may lead to an increased risk of bleeding caused by the interaction between blood and artificial surfaces and the use of anticoagulants. Patients previously treated with percutaneous cardiac or peripheral vascular stenting may be treated with clopidogrel and/or aspirin, leading to diffuse bleeding. In these cases, a surgical drain (10 French Jackson-Pratt drain, placed to bulb suction) is placed and kept until the drainage is serosanguinous and daily output has diminished (volume determined by surgeon preference). Graft ultrasonography is useful to evaluate for surgical perigraft hematoma. A large hematoma may compress the kidney or become infected and necessitate surgical washout.

A dreaded (but rare) intra-operative complication in a patient not adequately treated with neuromuscular blockade is the "scissoring" of the abdominal muscles, after retractors are taken out, leading to the kidney being pulled off its vascular pedicle or rupture of the vascular anastomosis and massive hemorrhage and possible graft loss. When this occurs, it is best to clamp the iliacs, remove the kidney, flush it, and re-implant it.

Hyperkalemia (*See* Chapter 16)

Oliguria

Oliguria as defined by decreased urine output (<500 mL/24 hours) is an indicator, together with increase in serum creatinine and potassium, of acute kidney injury. It is of utmost importance to address oliguria quickly in a post-transplant patient with previous normal urine output. The first management step should always be to administer bolus intravenous fluids to exclude prerenal azotemia as etiology. Consider invasive monitoring if the volemic status is questioned or if the patient has significant history of cardiac morbidity. Dialysis may be needed for symptomatic fluid overload.

Reasons for an abrupt decrease in urine output post-transplant can include graft thrombosis (discussed separately below). A slower decrease in urine output (coupled with an increase in creatinine) may be related to DGF and/or drug toxicity (usually from calcineurin inhibitors). Urine output and creatinine should normalize as serum drug levels become therapeutic. Oliguria is typically followed by a polyuric phase without a fall in serum creatinine, followed by normalization of both urine output and creatinine.

Graft Thrombosis
In the balance between bleeding and thrombosis, bleeding is the most favorable. Using blood transfusions, correction of coagulopathy, or return to the operating room to identify and repair the bleeding and evacuating the hematoma rarely puts the patient or the graft at risk. However, thrombosis of the transplanted kidney or the ipsilateral lower extremity may risk both the graft and the patient's leg. Graft thrombosis (venous thrombosis is more frequent than arterial thrombosis) can be confirmed by ultrasound and is an indication for emergent exploration to attempt to rescue the kidney. In the operating room, the presence and exact location of a thrombosis may be discovered. Renal vessels may need to be shortened in case they are kinked. Blood supply may be interrupted if the kidney undergoes torsion along its vascular axis. If identified quickly, blood flow may be re-established by repositioning the kidney and fixing it in a safe position. The iliac or renal vessels can be opened longitudinally, and a thrombus may be removed using Fogarty catheters. Most of the time, the kidney will not be salvageable and will have to be removed. A study from the University of Minnesota found that 15 of 933 (1.6%) grafts were lost to early vascular thrombosis (Matas et al., 2002).

Injuries on the recipient iliac artery may occur, most commonly from a vascular clamp placed during graft revascularization. Peripheral pulses should always be monitored post-transplant, and immediately examined with Doppler if physical exam changes or if the patient complains of unilateral pain or any other signs of compromised extremity.

Urine Leak
The reported frequency of urine leak varied between 0% and 9.3% of cases. Surgical technique may have an impact on leak frequency, with open (Leadbetter-Politano—two cystotomies) having a higher risk than the extravesical (Lich—only one cystotomy). The use of ureteral stents may have an impact on leak rate, but this remains controversial and may increase the risk of infectious complications. At UPMC, our urine leak frequency is less than 2%. Other factors contributing to the risk of urine leak include recipient age,

presence of multiple (inferior pole) arteries, acute rejection, or recipient bladder problems.

Symptoms of urine leak are usually early post-transplant and include fever, pain over graft, fluid leak from wound, persistent JP output (if placed), and increasing serum creatinine. Work-up of these patients should include abdominal imaging. A fluid collection may be drained percutaneously, and a fluid creatinine will give the diagnosis. A renal nuclear scan may be performed if frank fluid collection is not seen or is nonspecific, as can be the case if the kidney is placed intraperitoneally.

The treatment consists of surgical re-exploration if diagnosed early or high volume indicating a significant leak that will not heal with conservative measures. The majority of leaks can be treated with urinary tract stenting (percutaneous nephrostomy with stent placement) or prolonged Foley drainage.

Ureteral Obstruction

The frequency of ureteral obstruction is between 1% and 8.3%. Early ureteral obstruction is most likely related to compressing hematoma, edema, kinking, and blood clots. Late obstruction can result from fibrosis, ischemia, or acute rejection. The diagnosis is usually made by the work-up for a rising serum creatinine by hydronephrosis seen on ultrasonography. A Lasix washout renogram may be helpful to diagnose ureteral obstruction, but the most sensitive technique is antegrade nephrostogram, which has the benefit of decompressing the kidney, and eventually treats the obstruction with ureteral dilatation and stent placement. Infected kidneys must be externally drained. Only after the creatinine has returned to baseline and the infection has been adequately treated should definitive treatment be considered. If interventional therapy fails, then operative management depends on the stricture location. Distal strictures may be excised, with creation of a new vesiculoureteral anastomosis. More proximal strictures may be bypassed using a ureteroureterostomy to the native ureter.

Hemolytic Uremic Syndrome

Classical Hemolytic Uremic syndrome (HUS) is characterized by hemolytic anemia, thrombocytopenia, and renal impairment. The term thrombotic microangiopathy (TMA) is used interchangeably with HUS. Most often it occurs in children, and the typical etiology is *Escherichia coli* infection (O157:H7 serotype). Atypical HUS represents the 10% of cases that are not caused by the usual infectious agents; it has a poor prognosis, with 25% mortality and 50% renal dysfunction leading to end-stage renal disease.

Kidney transplant recipients may have recurrence of HUS, with very poor outcome, as reviewed by Ponticelli and Banfi (2006). Treatment consists of plasma infusions or plasmapheresis. High-dose IVIG and Rituximab have also been attempted, with unclear clinical benefit.

Patients with de novo post-transplant TMA have a better chance of graft salvage (about 80%) with plasmapheresis. It is estimated that 1% to 5% of kidney transplant recipients will be diagnosed with de novo post-transplant TMA. Risk factors include marginal donor kidneys, CMV infection, parvovirus B19 infection, or malignancy. The most important risk factors are the immunosuppressive drugs tacrolimus, cyclosporine, and also mTor inhibitors. The mechanisms for de novo TMA are poorly understood. Most commonly, de novo TMA occurs early but may also be seen up to 6 years post-transplant.

Rejection

With the advent of more effective immunosuppressive agents, the incidence of rejection episodes in kidney transplant recipients has fallen from 40% to 50 % in 1980s to less than 10% during the first year. Still, acute rejection is a potential risk factor for developing chronic allograft dysfunction and graft loss.

Rejection Types
There are three main types of clinical rejection:
1. Hyperacute rejection
2. Acute rejection—The two histologically defined types of acute rejection are:
   a. Acute cellular rejection
   b. Acute antibody-mediated rejection
3. Interstitial fibrosis/tubular atrophy (formerly chronic allograft nephropathy, formerly chronic rejection)

Hyperacute Rejection
Hyperacute rejection is caused by preformed DSAs, such as ABO isoagglutinins, anti-endothelial antibodies, and anti-HLA antibodies. It usually occurs anytime between the revascularization of the kidney to 48 hours post-transplantation, usually resulting in graft loss within the first hour. The diagnosis of hyperacute rejection is usually made intra-operatively when it presents immediately after reperfusion, as the kidney appears blue and flaccid and without blood flow. A biopsy would show thrombi occluding the small arteries and glomeruli and renal cortical necrosis. The transplanted kidney cannot be saved and must be removed once the diagnosis is confirmed. Most hyperacute rejection can be prevented by confirming a negative cross-match before surgery.

Acute Rejection
Acute rejection is defined as an acute deterioration in graft function associated with specific pathological changes in the allograft biopsy. It occurs usually within first year after transplant.

With current immunosuppressive drugs, signs and symptoms of acute rejection tend to be mild and may be completely asymptomatic. Most commonly, rejection is diagnosed by detecting an elevated serum creatinine and may or may not (usually acute rejection is asymptomatic) involve mild accompanying symptoms such as fever, pain at graft site, decreased urine output, and general malaise. The differential diagnosis must include graft dysfunction secondary to prerenal, renal, or postrenal causes like dehydration, drug toxicity, infection, recurrence of primary disease, or urinary obstruction. Ultimately, a histological assessment of the graft is required to confirm the diagnosis of acute rejection, most commonly via a percutaneous kidney biopsy. The two principal histological forms of acute rejection are acute cellular rejection (ACR), which is characterized by infiltration of the allograft by lymphocytes and other inflammatory cells and acute antibody-mediated rejection (AMR), which is characterized by identification of DSA in the recipients' serum in the presence of graft dysfunction and supported by immunohistological findings (including C4d-positive stains).

The Banff classification system not only provides current diagnostic categories for renal allograft biopsies but also helps in guiding strategies to treat acute rejection, depending on severity and type of rejection:

Category 1: Normal—A histologically normal biopsy.

Category 2: Antibody-mediated changes—This may be concurrent with categories 3 to 6. It results from documentation of circulating anti-donor antibody, C4d, and allograft pathology.

- Indeterminate AMR—C4d deposition without morphological evidence of active rejection
- Acute AMR
- Chronic active AMR

Category 3: Borderline changes—Suspicious for acute T-cell-mediated rejection. "Suspicious" for acute T-cell-mediated rejection (may coincide with categories 2, 5, and 6).

Category 4: T-cell-mediated rejection—This may be concurrent with categories 2, 5, and 6.

Category 5: Interstitial fibrosis and tubular atrophy, without evidence of any specific etiology. This used to be termed chronic allograft nephropathy.

Category 6: Other—This category consists of changes not thought to result from acute and/or chronic rejection. It includes chronic hypertension, calcineurin inhibitor toxicity, chronic obstruction, pyelonephritis, and viral infections.

Options for the treatment of established acute rejection include pulse steroids, antibodies (monoclonal or polyclonal), adjustment of baseline immunosuppression, and/or other therapies like plasmapheresis. Treatment depends on whether the rejection is ACR or AMR; severity of rejection chronic changes; presence of viral infections like BK, CMV, or EBV; or presence of bacterial infections or malignancies that would preclude from intensified immunosuppression.

At UPMC, we use the following protocol:

- Biopsy—Borderline changes
    - o 1–3 doses of steroid
- Biopsy—ACR Banff IA-IB
    - o 3 days of pulse steroids (Solu-medrol 500 mg daily)
    - o Augment the dose of tacrolimus and mycophenolate mofetil, if necessary.

- o In case of unfavorable clinical response or worsening graft function after three doses solu-medrol, we consider rebiopsy and if severity of rejection is same or worse, then we treat as steroid resistant rejection as discussed below.
- Biopsy—ACR II-III/ steroid-resistant rejection
  - o We use thymoglobulin at a daily doses of 1 mg/kg for 7 to 10 days; or
  - o Campath 1H 30 mg single dose; or
  - o Intravenous immune globulin (IVIG) 500 mg/kg/day (4 doses)
  - o No favorable response to this regimen; we will rebiopsy to make sure that AMR is not present. This includes repeat C4d staining and an analysis for DSAs.

Whenever Thymoglobulin or Campath is used, we put the patients on antiviral (valganciclovir) prophylaxis for 6 months and antifungal (nystatin) prophylaxis for 3 months.

- Biopsy—AMR either alone or in combination with cellular rejection
  - o We treat aggressively to remove or inhibit circulating anti-donor antibodies. We use plasmapheresis three times weekly with IVIG 100 mg/kg after each session. Steroid boluses are also used in certain cases with associated ACR. We check for DSA prior to initiating treatment and weekly during the treatment course.
  - o In acute AMR cases refractory to above treatment or recurrent AMR, Rituximab (an anti-CD20 antibody targeting B cells) is given as a one-time dose. In certain cases, bortezomib (a proteasome inhibitor) is also used.

Chronic Rejection

"Interstitial fibrosis and tubular atrophy, without evidence of any specific etiology" described in Category 5 of Banff classification is considered a preferred term, rather than chronic rejection or chronic allograft nephropathy. It is most common cause of death censored graft loss.

The clinical diagnosis is suggested by gradual deterioration of graft function, as manifested by a slowly rising plasma creatinine concentration, increasing proteinuria, and worsening hypertension; the diagnosis is confirmed pathologically with changes involving all parts of the renal parenchyma, including the blood vessels, glomeruli, interstitium, and tubules.

Once diagnosed, we consider reduction of calcineurin inhibitor dosage with or without addition of a non-nephrotoxic immunosuppressive agent and, if indicated, referred for evaluation for retransplantation.

Selected Reference

Ponticelli C, Banfi G. Thrombotic microangiopathy after kidney transplantation. *Transpl Int.* 2006;19(10):789–794.

Li EN, Silverman RP, Goldberg NH. Incisional hernia repair in renal transplantation patients. *Hernia.* 2005;9(3):231–237.

Matas AJ, Humar A, Gillingham KJ, Payne WD, Gruessner RWG, Kandaswamy R, Dunn DL, Najarian JS, Sutherland, DER. Five preventable causes of kidney graft loss in the 1990s: A single-center analysis. *Kid Internat.* 2002;62:704–714

Shapiro R. The transplant procedure. In: Shapiro R, Simmons RL, Starzl TE, eds. *Renal Transplantation* (p. 1) Stamford, CT: Appleton & Lange; 1998.

Chapter 19

Pancreas Transplantation

Peter Abrams, Mark Sturdevant, Abhinav Humar,
and Ron Shapiro

Introduction

Pancreas transplantation remains the optimal and most durable form of glucose management therapy for selected patients with complications from type I or type II diabetes mellitus (DM). A well-functioning solid-organ pancreas transplant establishes euglycemia in patients with advanced disease, delivering all of the well-established benefits of intensive glycemic control while eliminating the significant financial costs and quality-of-life impairments of continuous monitoring and administration of exogenous insulin. Novel strategies for immunosuppression, including induction therapy and rapid steroid withdrawal, have resulted in substantially lower rates of pancreas allograft rejection and improved graft survival over the past decade, confirming the role of pancreas transplantation in selected patients with complicated DM.

Indications for Pancreas Transplantation

Selected patients with severe and disabling complications from DM may be candidates for pancreas transplant alone (PTA), simultaneous pancreas-kidney transplant (SPK), or pancreas after kidney transplant (PAK). The majority of pancreas transplant recipients are uremic diabetics; therefore, SPK is the most commonly performed pancreas transplant operation. The two criteria for pancreas transplantation according to the American Diabetes Association are:

1. consistent failure of intensive-based therapy to establish reasonable glycemic control and prevent secondary complications; and
2. incapacitating clinical and emotional problems with exogenous insulin therapy.

In the absence of meeting the first criterion, the second criterion requires careful clinical judgment in deciding whether a patient is an appropriate pancreas transplant candidate. Patients who meet the second criterion generally have frequent admissions for DM ketoacidosis or have episodes of hypoglycemic unawareness.

Contraindications to Pancreas Transplantation

Apart from contraindications that are similar to those for other solid-organ transplants, historically the most specific relative contraindication to pancreas transplantation has been the diagnosis of type II DM involving insulin resistance. Each potential pancreas candidate must be thoroughly evaluated for the presence of insulin resistance, which theoretically would (but, in practice, may not) inhibit or impede a pancreas allograft from achieving normal glycemic control. Although single-center data have demonstrated good results in type II diabetic patients, not all centers will consider them for pancreas transplantation.

Evaluation for Pancreas Transplantation

The goals of the pretransplant evaluation are to determine overall suitability for pancreas transplantation and to identify risk factors that increase the risk of patient death, graft loss, or significant morbidity. Determining which type of pancreas transplant to perform and careful patient selection are essential to optimize the potential benefits of pancreas transplantation. Patients with disabling DM and intact native renal or renal allograft function may be considered for PTA or PAK, respectively. Patients with brittle DM who have varying degrees of Chronic Kidney Disease (CKD) Glomerular Filtration Rate (GFR <40 mL/min) are considered for SPK. Risk factors in this patient population include advancing age, obesity, adverse psychosocial factors, pre-existing cardiovascular disease, chronic viral illness (Hepatitis C, HIV), gastrointestinal disorders (peptic ulcer disease and pancreatitis), chronic obstructive pulmonary disease, and previously treated malignancies.

Most patients suffering from DM die of cardiovascular complications. Accelerated atherosclerosis and associated thrombogenesis contribute significantly to cardiovascular morbidity. Cardiac morbidity remains a significant challenge in pancreas recipients. Candidates with coronary artery disease are therefore evaluated prior to transplantation through consultation with cardiologists and even cardiac surgeons. As at least one-third of asymptomatic patients with type I DM and ESRD will have significant coronary artery disease on angiography, and echocardiography alone appears insufficient in reliably detecting significant coronary disease in these high-risk patients. Cardiac catheterization is often part of the routine preoperative evaluation for all pancreas candidates older than 45 years of age . Furthermore, there is historical evidence to suggest that detection of asymptomatic coronary artery disease in uremic diabetic patients and revascularization prior to transplantation may lead to improved outcomes in terms of cardiac morbidity and mortality.

As pancreas allograft thrombosis remains the leading non-immunological cause of graft loss after pancreas transplantation, it is advised that candidates be evaluated for hypercoagulable states (HCS), especially the more common disorders, including Factor V Leiden. Although the presence of a HCS would not necessarily preclude consideration for pancreas transplantation, long-term post-transplant anti-coagulation management would likely be required.

Selected References

Gruessner AC & Sutherland DE. Pancreas transplant outcomes for United States (US) and non-US cases as reported to the United Network for Organ Sharing (UNOS) and the International Pancreas Transplant Registry (IPTR) as of June 2004. *Clin Transplant* 2005;19:433–455.

White SA, Shaw JA, & Sutherland DER. Pancreas transplantation. *Lancet* 2009;373:1808–1817.

Chapter 20

Anesthetic Management of Pancreatic Transplant Recipients

Ibtesam A. Hilmi, Ali R. Abdullah, and Raymond M. Planinsic

Introduction: Peri-operative care and anesthetic management of pancreatic transplant recipients (PTx) is very much dependent on the presence or absence of comorbidities and the severity of end-organ damages that are caused by the chronic hyperglycemic state.

Pre-Operative Evaluation and Preparation for Pancreatic Transplantation

Diabetic patients who are evaluated for possible pancreatic transplantation usually undergo the following evaluation process:

1. CVS evaluation: Examination for the existence and the extent of coronary artery disease, hypertension, and peripheral vascular disease. A thorough medical history and clinical examination are made. In addition, it is advisable to obtain further diagnostic tests such as exercise stress test (or dobutamine stress ECHO) and/or coronary angiography and bilateral carotid Doppler—especially for patients with peripheral vascular disease.

2. Renal evaluation: The existence and the extent of renal involvement can be determined by the presence of microalbuminuria, estimation of GFR, and serum creatinine level. In case of the presence of ESRD in diabetic patients, a combined kidney-pancreas transplant may be considered.

3. Neurological Evaluation: Involvement of somatic and autonomic nervous system should be documented and properly evaluated by neurological team.

4. Evaluation of the Musculoskeletal involvement: This included the presence of joint stiffness especially cervical spine and temperomandibular joint, as involvement of these joints may affect airway management during the peri-operative period.

5. Blood glucose control: This could be evaluated properly by measuring the glycosylated HbA1c, which is not affected by short-term fluctuation

in blood glucose. Chronically elevated HbA1c not only reflects poorly controlled hyperglycemia but can predict the presence of diabetic vasculopathy.

Intra-Operative Monitoring

The type of monitoring during PTx is very much dependent on the presence of comorbidity and the experience of the anesthesia providers with a certain type of monitoring technology.

The pancreatic transplant surgery by itself is associated with minimal fluid shift and minimal blood loss; however, the recipients may have complicated medical history, and managing them could be a challenging task. In recipients who do not suffer from serious CVS or renal diseases, invasive blood pressure monitoring typically with radial artery catherization is all that is required along with peripheral intravenous access. Central venous access and/or pulmonary artery catheter, transesophageal echocardiography may be needed in certain pancreatic recipients or in patients who are receiving combined kidney–pancreas transplant and present with more complicated cardiovascular disease.

Premedications

Metoclopramide and H_2 blocker should be considered in patients with autonomic gastroparesis. In preparation for intra-operative infusion of immune induction agent (alemtuzamab, Campath-1H®, Bayer HealthCare Pharmaceuticals Formerly Berlex Laboratories Inc.), 1 g methyl prednisolone, 50 mg diphenhydramine, 650 mg acetaminophen, and 20 mg famotidine are routinely given before the start of anesthesia and surgery. Campath should be started after the induction of anesthesia and establishment of the required monitoring because it has the potential of causing serious complications such as hypotension, bronchospasm, and even anaphylactic reaction.

Intra-Operative Management

General anesthesia is preferred over regional anesthesia for pancreas transplant. Diabetic patients may be more prone to develop neuronal injury by local anesthetic-induced neurotoxicity. In diabetic patients, the risk of infection and developing an epidural abscess is higher than in non-diabetic patients. As with all transplant recipients, this risk will be higher because these patients will receive powerful immunosuppressant medications.

Rapid-sequence induction is preferable in pancreatic transplant recipients due to the high risk of passive regurgitation and aspiration. If difficult air way or difficult intubation is suspected then awake fiberoptic intubation will be the safest option. The choice of the induction agent, dose, and rate of injection depend on presence of comorbidity and the preference of the anesthesiologist. The choice of the muscle relaxant depends on the presence of adequate renal function; in the case of end-stage renal disease (ESRD), cisatracurium may be a better choice, but rocuronium and vacuronium are both metabolized primarily by the liver and can be used safely during PTx. Narcotics can be used with some reservations if the patients have nephropathy because some narcotics have active metabolites, such as miperidine and morphine, that are excreted by the kidney. However, fentanyl and remifantinal can be used safely. Surgery takes approximately 2 to 4 hours, and the main goal of anesthesia is to provide absolute hemodynamic stability by whatever means necessary to ensure adequate blood flow to all vital organs, including the pancreas. The choice of vasopressor agent depends on the cardiovascular condition of the recipients, but beta-agonists are preferable over alpha-agonist to avoid direct vasoconstriction.

Arterial blood gas sampling is monitored hourly and more frequently (20–30 minutes) after reperfusion, for early monitoring of pancreatic function by the response of the blood glucose to insulin secretion.

During emergence from anesthesia, it is important to control the heart rate and blood pressure and preferably to use short-acting beta-blocker (esmolol) and/or nitroglycerine, which may help in ameliorating the sympathetic response to emergence and extubation.

Post-Operative Care

Most of these patients were admitted to the intensive care unit (ICU) to ensure an accurate blood glucose monitoring as an indicator of pancreatic allograft function. Other indications for postoperative ICU admission are related to the presence of serious cardiovascular, renal, autonomic neuropathy, or respiratory disease or the occurrences of unexpected intra-operative complications. The post-operative pain is usually managed by patient-controlled analgesia with careful monitoring resulting from compromised ventilatory response to hypoxia and hypercapnia.

Chapter 21

Surgical Techniques of Pancreas Transplantation

Peter Abrams, Mark Sturdevant, Ron Shapiro, and Abhinav Humar

Organ Procurement and Back-Table Preparation

Performing a successful pancreas transplant requires meticulous attention to detail and technical mastery in all phases of organ recovery, preparation, and implantation. The rapid en bloc technique for combined liver-pancreas recovery has already been well described and validated by its use in thousands of successful procurements by the Pittsburgh group and others. The deceased donor en bloc pancreatic specimen includes the pancreas, most of the duodenum, and spleen. In 18% to 22% of organ donors, a replaced right hepatic artery (RHA) originates from the superior mesenteric artery (SMA). A replaced RHA has historically been considered a contraindication to the separate procurement of the liver and pancreas. It is now the practice of many pancreatic transplant centers to utilize the pancreas after dividing the SMA distal to the take-off of the replaced RHA as long as adequate length can be achieved to preserve inflow to the inferior pancreaticoduodenal artery (IPDA).

Careful inspection of the pancreas is important to determine whether traumatic injury, surgical damage, or poor allograft quality secondary to fibrosis or fatty infiltration would preclude its further consideration for transplantation. The arterial blood supply to the pancreas allograft includes the splenic artery (SA), which supplies the body and tail of the pancreas, and proximal SMA, which supplies the pancreatic head through the IPDA. It is critical to confirm that the IPDA has been preserved to proceed with transplantation. It is expected that the gastroduodenal artery (GDA) will have been ligated and divided at its origin by the procurement team. Venous drainage of the pancreas allograft includes a short segment of portal vein just above the confluence of the splenic vein and superior mesenteric vein (SMV). The absence of even a small segment of portal vein should not be considered an absolute contraindication to transplantation, as mobilization of the allograft venous confluence, use of a venous extension graft, and mobilization of the recipient external iliac vein are usually adequate for addressing the lack of significant portal vein length.

Once a complete back-table preparation of the pancreas has been performed, the allograft should be flushed again with chilled preservation solution. It is prudent to use fresh solution to avoid the infusion of small particles of tissue or fat into the allograft. Flushing allows the surgeon to evaluate the vascular reconstructions and identify any overlooked vessels that require ligation. If the allograft has been procured properly, the efflux from the venous extension graft should at this point be non-bloody. After flushing confirms a well-perfused pancreas allograft with sound vascular reconstructions, the organ is ready to be implanted.

Implantation

There are many options in terms of techniques for implanting the pancreas allograft. These variations include different types of skin incision, orientation of the pancreas in the abdomen, systemic or portal venous drainage, and bladder or enteric drainage of the exocrine pancreas. From 2004 through 2008, enteric drainage was the most frequently used technique in U.S. transplant centers for all three types of pancreas transplants and is the preferred technique at the University of Pittsburgh[1]. The use of portal venous drainage has declined in the past decade. For enterically drained pancreas transplants, reported rates of portal drainage are 21% of SPK transplants, 17% of PAK transplants, and 15% of PTA transplants. This section provides a concise description of the implantation procedure performed most commonly at our center, as a discussion of the advantages and disadvantages of each technical variation is outside the scope of this chapter.

After a lower midline incision is performed, attention is turned to the right lower quandrant, with exposure of the right common and external iliac artery and vein. When using systemic venous drainage, the right internal iliac vein may be ligated and divided to mobilize the distal external iliac vein for the anastomosis. The venous anastomosis is performed first. The pancreas is oriented in a "head-down" orientation so that the superior aspect of the pancreas is facing posterior, the tail of the pancreas is pointing cephalad, and the duodenum is caudad. The portal vein, with or without a venous conduit, is anastomosed end-to-side to the distal external iliac vein. The artery is anastomosed either end-to-side to the proximal external iliac artery, or end-to-end to the internal iliac artery. After completion of the vascular anastomoses, the allograft is reperfused. A normal pancreas allograft will reperfuse in relatively uniform fashion, turning a tan-pink color almost immediately. Hemostasis is achieved following reperfusion. Finally, exocrine drainage is achieved. A mid- to distal jejunal segment of small bowel is identified for the duodenojejunostomy anastomosis. After ensuring there is no tension on the mesentery as the loop of jejunum is delivered to the donor duodenal segment in the right lower quadrant, a two-layer, hand-sewn, side-to-side bowel anastomosis is performed in the usual fashion. Some surgeons will place drains prior to abdominal closure.

Post-Operative Management After Pancreas Transplantation

General surgical principles guide the management of the pancreas transplant recipient in the immediate post-operative period. Routine postsurgical care includes admission to the intensive care unit (ICU) for the first 1 to 2 days, frequent measurement of vital signs, daily laboratory values, nasogastric decompression usually for the first few post-operative days, incentive spirometry, Foley catheter drainage, patient-controlled analgesia for pain management, and pneumatic compression stockings for DVT prophylaxis.

Management of Intravascular Volume

Intravenous fluid replacement commonly consists of half-normal saline and is titrated based on urine output. A drop in urine output related to inadequate filling pressures should be treated with a crystalloid or colloid bolus. Many pancreas transplant recipients are chronically hypovolemic prior to transplant partly because of fluid shifts caused by poor glycemic control, and adequate volume resuscitation can commonly extend into the post-operative management period. In terms of maintaining electrolyte balance, most transplant centers have protocol order sets for acute replacement of potassium and magnesium. Bladder-drained (BD) pancreas transplant recipients can lose significant amounts of sodium bicarbonate (1–3L/day) from pancreatic exocrine and duodenal mucosal secretions into the urine. Adequate volumes of oral and intravenous sodium bicarbonate are administered to prevent hyperchloremic metabolic acidosis, dehydration, and orthostasis.

Optimization of Cardiovascular Function

Maintenance of appropriate allograft perfusion pressure is critical to successful outcomes in pancreas transplantation. In "high-risk" recipients, invasive hemodynamic monitoring may be indicated for assessment of cardiac filling pressures. To avoid pulmonary congestion and heart failure, fluid challenges in these diabetic patients must be administered with caution. Hypertensive crises are to be avoided, as high pressures can lead to bleeding in addition to serious cardiac complications. Conversely, hypotension secondary to hypovolemia causes inadequate left ventricular filling pressures, decreased cardiac output, and allograft hypoperfusion, increasing the risk of pancreas allograft thrombosis.

Maintenance of Euglycemia

Intensive glycemic monitoring is performed to maintain blood glucose levels between 80 and 120 mg/dL to avoid allograft beta-cell toxicity, using continuous intravenous insulin therapy as necessary. The intravenous insulin is commonly weaned over the first 1 to 2 post-operative days. A sudden elevation in blood glucose may indicate allograft thrombosis. After acute hyperglycemia has been confirmed and nonsurgical causes expeditiously excluded, an emergent Doppler ultrasound study should be performed to examine allograft arterial and venous flow. If there is any significant abnormality in flow, then a surgical re-exploration to evaluate for thrombosis is indicated. A thrombosed pancreas allograft should be removed without delay.

Post-Operative Anticoagulation

Because of the low-flow microcirculation within the pancreas allograft, at our center enoxaparin therapy is initiated at 0.5 mg/kg once or twice per day and is continued until day of discharge. All recipients receive aspirin 81 mg/day starting on the first post-operative day. Other options include use of continuous intravenous low-dose heparin during the immediate post-operative period.

Post-Operative Anylase and Lipase

The presence of elevated levels of amylase and lipase is expected and likely related to ischemia-reperfusion injury. Elevations in amylase and lipase in the immediate post-operative period in general are self-limited and do not require any additional work-up; occasionally, for significant elevations in amylase and lipase, subcutaneous octreotide is administered for a few days.

Post-Operative Renal Function in the Pancreas Recipient

Assessment and management of renal function after pancreas transplantation depends on whether a kidney transplant has simultaneously been performed. Although pancreas transplant alone (PTA) and pancreas after kidney transplant (PAK) recipients should have close to normal renal function in the peri-operative period, simultaneous pancreas-kidney transplant (SPK) patients may require dialysis both before and after transplant. When a candidate with marginal renal function is admitted to the hospital to undergo a pancreas transplant, pre-operative dialysis should be performed only for urgent indications such as hyperkalemia and/or moderate-to-severe volume overload, in order to avoid prolonged cold ischemia time. In patients with previous kidney transplants who undergo PAK, changes in urine output in the post-operative period are expected and usually result from volume shifts and ATN-related renal allograft injury. Rejection of the pre-existing kidney allograft in the pancreas transplant peri-operative period is unlikely, as the degree of immunosuppression at this time is typically much higher than the maintenance regimen for the kidney transplant.

Immunosuppression

Acute cellular rejection (ACR) is the most important factor contributing to graft loss in recipients who undergo a technically successful pancreas transplant. Drug regimens designed to prevent ACR in pancreas transplant recipients historically have involved induction with lymphocyte-depleting or nondepleting antibody and triple maintenance therapy with a calcineurin inhibitor, antimetabolite, and corticosteroids. The introduction of tacrolimus (FK 506, Prograf) and myco-phenolate mofetil (MMF, Cellcept) in the mid-1990s significantly improved the quality of maintenance immunosuppression by lowering rejection rates. The incidence of pancreas rejection varies according to transplant type: it is highest in nonuremic PTA recipients, followed by posturemic PAK recipients, and lowest in uremic SPK recipients. Accordingly, levels of immunosuppression are required to be highest in PTA recipients and slightly lower in PAK and SPK recipients. Diversion from general guidelines for level of immunosuppression is required under many circumstances, particularly in high-risk for rejection cohorts such as very young recipients, African-American recipients, high panel-reactive antibody titer recipients, and retransplant recipients, all of whom require more potent immunosuppression.

According to national data, patients undergoing PTA, PAK, and SPK between 2004 and 2008 received some form of antibody induction therapy in 88%, 80%, and 84% of cases, respectively. Although there has been wide variation in the type of antibody induction therapy used by transplant centers, induction therapy consisted of lymphocyte-depleting polyclonal anti-thymocyte globulin (Thymoglobulin) in 50% to 60% of cases, whereas 9% to 15% received the depleting monoclonal alemtuzumab (Campath 1H). Other induction agents included Atgam, OKT3, and non-depleting monoclonal daclizumab (Zenapax—now no longer available) and basiliximab (Simulect).

A significant variety of maintenance immunosuppression protocols have been used by pancreas centers in the United States, with the majority of programs using tacrolimus and MMF with or without other agents, and a growing trend of adding (or replacing other agents with) sirolimus (Rapamune) and minimizing or eliminating steroids. Between 2004 and 2008, a de novo steroid-free maintenance regimen was used in one-third of all SPK and PAK recipients. The most commonly used maintenance immunosuppression regimens for PTA recipients in 2007 at 1-year post-transplant were tacrolimus and steroids (27.3%), tacrolimus in combination with MMF and steroids (22%), tacrolimus and MMF without steroids (18%), and tacrolimus in combination with MMF and sirolimus (10.7%). For PAK recipients in 2007, 45% of patients at 1-year post-transplant were receiving tacrolimus along with MMF and steroids, whereas 24% were taking tacrolimus and MMF without steroids, and 7.8% were taking tacrolimus and MMF in combination with sirolimus. For SPK recipients in 2007, 53% were receiving triple immunosuppression with tacrolimus, MMF, and steroids, whereas 20% received tacrolimus and MMF without steroids.

Infectious Disease Management

The prevention of infection in these highly immunosuppressed patients requires a multi-faceted approach to address potential bacterial, fungal, and viral pathogens. All pancreas transplant recipients receive a 3- to 5-day course of broad spectrum antibiotics and antifungal prophylaxis in the peri-operative period. The majority of transplant centers will start oral nystatin, trimethoprim-sulfamethoxazole and some regimen for anti-cytomegalovirus (CMV) prophylaxis in the early post-operative period. Patients who are high-risk CMV-mismatch (i.e., donor-seropositive and recipient-seronegative) should receive a more prolonged course of anti-CMV prophylaxis.

Surgical site infections in pancreas transplant recipients have been historically reported in up to 30% of cases. Clinical signs of infection include wound dehiscence, bacterial peritonitis, intra-abdominal abscess, urinary tract infection, pneumonia, and systemic sepsis. Urinary tract infection in BD pancreas recipients is nearly universal. A high index of suspicion for infection, particularly in the first 4 to 6 weeks following pancreas transplantation, is critical for early diagnosis and timely definitive treatment.

Cytomegalovirus infection can manifest as a systemic viral syndrome or disease localized to the pancreas allograft. The typical clinical presentation involves acute pancreatitis with gastrointestinal bleeding. In the setting of acute CMV infection, it may be difficult for even well-trained transplant pathologists to exclude a concomitant episode of acute cellular rejection. The standard treatment for pancreas allograft CMV infection involves reduction of immunosuppression and initiation of intensive anti-CMV therapy.

The incidence of post-transplant lymphoproliferative disorder (PTLD) in pancreas transplant recipients has historically been reported between 2.2% and 12%. Often representing a complication of Epstein-Barr virus (EBV) infection in the setting of a suppressed immune system, PTLD can also manifest systemically or focally within the pancreas allograft. In pancreas transplant recipients, PTLD appears to be more aggressive with a worse prognosis compared to liver or kidney transplant recipients, with a higher stage at presentation and more bone marrow involvement. Cessation or marked reduction of immunosuppression achieves an adequate therapeutic response in many patients. Treatment of nonresponders can involve multiple modalities including anti-B cell therapy with Rituximab and/or chemotherapy; clinical outcomes after treatment are variable. It is critical to exclude severe acute rejection of the pancreas allograft before making the diagnosis of PTLD, as management of rejection involves escalation of immunosuppression rather than reduction.

Post-Transplant Monitoring of Pancreas Allograft Function

Monitoring of pancreas allograft endocrine function is achieved mainly by serial measurement of fasting blood glucose concentrations as well as C-peptide and glycosylated hemoglobin levels. The development of a mild-to-moderate degree of insulin resistance is not uncommon in the first 2 to 3 months following pancreas transplantation and can usually be successfully treated by tapering maintenance steroid therapy. Measuring serum amylase and lipase levels evaluates the exocrine function of the pancreas allograft and tends to be a relatively sensitive but nonspecific means of assessing the inflammatory status of the pancreas. In contrast to the management of elevated amylase and lipase levels in the immediate post-transplant period, detection of a sudden increase in these enzymes in the intermediate post-transplant period (i.e., within 4 weeks to 6 months) may indicate the presence of complications including infection, toxicity, reflux-related pancreatitis, abscess formation, or possible rejection and requires further medical evaluation.

Complications of Pancreas Transplantation

Despite advances in surgical technique, more than 10% of all pancreas allografts are lost because of technical reasons[2]. Slightly more than half of technical failures manifest as thrombosis of the allograft. Other causes include infection, pancreatitis, anastomotic leak, and bleeding. Rates of infection, leak, and bleeding are similar for enteric drainage and BD recipients. In contrast, allograft pancreatitis occurs more frequently in BD recipients. In SPK recipients, technical failure remains the most common cause of allograft loss. For PTA recipients, technical failure is the second most common cause of allograft loss, with rejection remaining the most common cause. Retrospective multivariate analysis of a large number of pancreas transplants performed at a single center has identified recipient obesity (body mass index > 30) and prolonged cold ischemia times (>24 hours) as important risk factors for technical failure.

Pancreas allograft thrombosis remains a significant clinical problem, with a reported incidence ranging from 5% to 13%. Various strategies of anticoagulation are used by different transplant centers in the immediate post-operative period to minimize the risk of allograft thrombosis, making bleeding a relatively common post-transplant complication. Fortunately, the impact of re-exploration for hemorrhage on allograft function and recipient mortality appears to be minimal. It is critical to evacuate hematoma surrounding the allograft in a timely fashion, as secondary infection may become a significant issue complicating post-operative hemorrhage in the early post-operative period.

Anastomotic leak following pancreas transplantation remains a common complication. Many different strategies have been attempted to address exocrine drainage of the pancreas allograft, including polymer injection of the pancreatic duct and open peritoneal drainage, both resulting in high rates of pancreatic fistula formation. With the two most accepted techniques for exocrine drainage involving bladder-drainage and enteric-drainage, the reported rate of anastomotic leak remains 9% to 14% in single-center experiences. Early post-transplant leaks occur secondary to technical reasons involving the transplant operation or donor procurement, including prolonged cold ischemia time, underappreciated duodenal trauma, post-reperfusion pancreatitis, and intra-abdominal infections. Late anastomotic leaks (i.e., occurring more than 3 months after transplant) occur more rarely, with a 2.5% incidence reported by the University of Minnesota group, and appear to be related to nonsurgical factors including ACR and CMV infection.

The presentation of pancreas recipients with anastomotic leak typically involves leukocytosis, elevated amylase and lipase levels, with a clinical exam significant for abdominal pain and tenderness. A CT scan is performed to confirm the presence of a fluid collection usually with associated inflammatory changes in surrounding soft tissues. Treatment of both early and late anastomotic leak requires surgical exploration in the presence of diffuse peritonitis or uncontrolled sepsis and may require allograft pancreatectomy, whereas conservative management with percutaneous drainage of collections and intravenous antibiotics can be used successfully in hemodynamically stable recipients with localized signs and symptoms.

The incidence of pancreas allograft loss following early anastomotic leak from a BD pancreas can exceed 20%, with a reported mortality rate of 7%. The allograft loss rate after early anastomotic leak from an enterically drained pancreas is higher, at 55%, with a mortality of 18%. Graft loss rates are similar following late anatomic leaks; however, mortality appears to be considerably lower.

Management of Pancreas Allograft Rejection

Episodes of pancreas allograft ACR are most likely to occur between 3 and 12 months following transplantation. Achieving timely diagnosis of pancreas ACR remains a challenge, as the typical accompanying signs and symptoms are nonspecific. Clinical presentations suggestive of ACR in pancreas transplant recipients include fever, tenderness over the allograft, abdominal pain, ileus, hematuria (for BD transplants), and swelling of the pancreas allograft. Laboratory findings during pancreas allograft ACR can include elevated serum amylase and lipase levels or decreased urinary amylase levels (for BD) on consecutive measurements. Elevated blood glucose levels are a relatively late manifestation of ACR that implies ongoing severe rejection with the strong possibility of allograft loss. For PAK and PTA recipients, the diagnosis of ACR is made definitively only by pancreas biopsy. For SPK recipients, where the kidney and pancreas have been transplanted from the same donor, the monitoring of serum creatinine appears to be a reliable means of detecting both kidney and pancreas ACR. Rejection of the SPK pancreas allograft in the absence of concomitant kidney allograft rejection with no change in the baseline serum creatinine is possible but not common.

The standard technique for pancreas allograft biopsy involves percutaneous biopsy under ultrasound or CT guidance. A series of 232 pancreas transplant biopsies under ultrasound guidance by an experienced pancreas transplant center demonstrated a complication rate of 2.6%, with three cases of intra-abdominal bleeding, and single episodes of gross hematuria, allograft pancreatitis, and severe pain requiring inpatient management.

In contrast to the treatment of ACR in kidney transplant recipients involving steroid monotherapy, the majority of rejection episodes involving pancreas allografts require more potent immunosuppression, usually involving corticosteroids and lymphocyte-depleting antibody in combination. From analysis of the SRTR (Scientific Registry of Transplant Recipients) database, the treatment of ACR in PTA recipients transplanted in 2007 involved corticosteroids and depleting antibody in 94.6% and 54.1% of cases, respectively. Treatment of ACR in PAK recipients involved corticosteroids in 85% of cases and antibody in 73% of cases (the majority of centers using anti-thymocyte globulin). Treatment of ACR in SPK recipients involved corticosteroids in 67% of cases and antibody in 51% of cases.

Current Outcomes of Pancreas Transplantation

Patient Survival

Although there is no unanimity of opinion, it appears that the well-established benefits of pancreas transplantation lead to a significant survival advantage in well-selected recipients. Rates of patient survival over the past decade have constantly improved, now exceeding 95% at 1 year post-transplant for all three types of pancreas transplants. Patient survival rates remain greater than 90% for all three types over the first 3 years post-transplant. The 5- and 10-year unadjusted patient survival rates are significantly higher for SPK (87% and 70%, respectively) and PTA (89% and 73%, respectively) recipients, compared to PAK recipients (84% and 65%, respectively). Actuarial 15-year patient survival remains 59% for PTA recipients, 56% for SPK recipients, and 42% for PAK recipients. Death of the recipient with a functioning graft remains the most common cause of graft loss (53%) after 10 years, followed by chronic rejection (33%).

There does not appear to be a substantial survival advantage after SPK compared to living-donor kidney transplant recipients in age-matched patients with type 1 Diabetes Mellitus (DM) over the long term. Similarly, it is not clear whether SPK recipients older than age 50 years gain any survival advantage over age-matched type 1 DM recipients receiving a deceased-donor kidney transplant. A recent analysis of the OPTN/UNOS database demonstrated improved renal allograft and patient survival despite inferior pancreas allograft survival in type 1 DM patients undergoing living-donor kidney transplantation followed by cadaveric pancreas transplantation compared to well-matched SPK recipients.

Graft Survival

Optimal longevity in terms of graft survival is achieved with SPK transplantation starting at 1 year post-transplant, with 1-year and 10-year pancreas graft survival rates of 86% and 53%, respectively. Long-term graft function of PAK recipients remains significantly better than PTA recipients, though this difference has become less pronounced in recent years. Unadjusted 1-year graft survival for PAK and PTA were similar at 77% and 81%, respectively, but gradually differentiate over the long term, with 10-year graft survival of 35% and 26%, respectively. The differences in longevity of graft function are explained mainly by significantly higher rates of allograft rejection and immunological graft loss in PTA and PAK recipients compared to SPK recipients. Reported graft loss rates at 1 year post-transplant was 2% for SPK recipients but 6% for PTA and PAK recipients. Immunological graft loss rates between PTA and PAK recipients remain similar over the short term, but at 3 years post-transplant PTA rates of graft loss become significantly higher than PAK.

Impact on Quality of Life

Although it is not straightforward to make generalized statements about improvements in quality of life after pancreas transplantation, as quality-of-life parameters are highly subjective and often confounded by complications of DM that are too advanced to be reversed, it is clear that the elimination of continuous blood glucose measurements, insulin injections and constraints on dietary intake represents a substantial improvement in overall quality of daily living. It remains (at least in the minds of some) unresolved, however, whether these significant benefits can potentially be outweighed by the impositions of immunosuppression management, treatment of rejection, complications of surgery, or financial challenges related to transplantation.

Impact on Diabetic Retinopathy, Nephropathy, and Neuropathy

The long-term impact of pancreas transplantation on the main complications of type 1 DM (e.g., retinopathy, nephropathy, and neuropathy) remains unclear because of an absence of large-scale and well-controlled long-term studies and because pancreas transplantation occurs late in the course of complicated DM. It is well established that more than 75% of patients diagnosed with type 1 DM as adults will develop retinopathy after 10 years. In this adult population with retinopathy, one-third of patients will demonstrate proliferative retinopathy, and approximately 40% will develop blindness after 3 years. After pancreas transplantation, retinopathy can progress in 10% to 35% of recipients with clinically unstable ophthalmic disease. Additionally, eye disease unassociated with type 1 DM, including cataracts, may also progress secondary to steroid use.

Nephropathy associated with type 1 DM results from accumulation of extracellular matrix proteins in the renal mesangium, glomerular and tubular basement membranes, and interstitium. After pancreas transplantation, the establishment of euglycemia can halt the progression of DM glomerulopathy but will not commonly cause regression. In patients with type 1 DM who undergo kidney transplant alone, experienced pathologists can detect morphological changes on allograft biopsy consistent with diabetic nephropathy as early as the first 2 to 3 months post-transplant. It has been reported that patients undergoing SPK will demonstrate diabetic nephropathy changes in the renal allograft to a much lesser extent or sometimes not at all.

Improvements in type 1 DM-related neuropathy have been reported in the literature following pancreas transplantation. These improvements can be subtle, and there is little evidence that recipients with advanced neuropathy have significant symptomatic improvement post-transplant. Overall, pancreas transplantation remains a legitimate modality for select patients with type 1 or type 2 DM with severe and disabling end-organ dysfunction.

Selected References

Corry RJ, Chakrabarti P, Shapiro R, et al. Comparison of enteric versus bladder drainage in pancreas transplantation. *Transplant Proc* 2001;33:1647.

Humar A, Ramcharan T, Kandaswamy R, Gruessner RW, Gruessner AC, & s Sutherland DE. Technical failures after pancreas transplants: why grafts fail and the risk factors—a multivariate analysis. *Transplantation* 2004;78(8):1188–1192.

Chapter 22

Islet Cell Transplantation

Ely M. Sebastian, Abhinav Humar, and Martin Wijkstrom

The first human islet allograft transplant was performed at the University of Minnesota in 1974. In 1977, the first successful total pancreatectomy and simultaneous islet autotransplantation was performed; the patient died 6 years later from unrelated causes. The first two successful total pancreatectomies and simultaneous heterotopic segmental pancreas autotransplants were reported in 1978; at that time, one patient had a functioning graft 3 years post-transplant and the second was lost to follow-up. In 1980, Largiader et al. were the first to report insulin independence in a type 1 diabetic (T1DM) recipient after an islet allotransplant and simultaneous kidney transplant. This patient underwent an intrasplenic transplant of pancreatic microfragments prepared from a 2.5-year-old donor. That patient became insulin independent at 8 months post-transplant while taking prednisone at a daily dose of 20 mg. In 1990, University of Pittsburgh reported insulin independence after combined solid-organ-islet transplant. Nine patients with surgical diabetes from upper-abdominal exenteration including total pancreatectomy were transplanted with a single-donor islet allotransplant. In 1993, the University of Minnesota demonstrated sustained insulin independence in two patients with T1DM after transplantation of unpurified islets from a single adult donor. In the following years, the average 1-year insulin independence rate was about 10%.

A landmark clinical trial reported by the group at the University of Alberta in Edmonton in 2000 in the *New England Journal of Medicine* marked a turning point in the history of islet transplantation. Of seven patients receiving islets from two to four donors, seven were insulin independent at 1 year using a steroid-free immunosuppressive regimen consisting of anti-interleukin (IL)-2 receptor antagonist induction and maintenance with sirolimus and low-dose tacrolimus. This study established safety and efficacy of islet allotransplantation as a treatment option for T1DM patients. Although this initial study showed proof-of-concept by correcting hyperglycemia and maintaining recipients insulin-free for 1 year, the 5-year follow-up clearly indicated that graft function was lost, or significantly reduced over time, with less than 10% of the patients remaining insulin-independent. Reasons for delayed graft loss are multifactorial and can be attributed to a combination of factors including allograft rejection, recurrent auto-immunity, diabetogenic side effects of immunosuppression, possible immunosuppression-associated detrimental effects of islet neogenesis, islet mass loss from ischemia-reperfusion injury and/or to instant blood-mediated inflammatory reaction, and unfavorable implant site.

Islet transplants can also be performed simultaneously with, or after, a kidney or other solid-organ transplant. Most common, however, is islet transplants alone in T1DM patients with hypoglycemia unawareness or auto islet transplantation in patients with severe chronic pancreatitis undergoing total pancreatectomy for the treatment of pain. The most recent Collaborative Islet Transplant Registry (CITR) has compiled results of more than 800 islet allotransplants from 1999 to 2008 (81% of transplants were performed in North America; the remaining 19% in the rest of the world). At most, a total of 32 centers participated in CITR, but several centers are no longer active following the report of poor long-term graft function.

Indications

Islet allotransplantation is an alternative to whole-organ pancreas transplantation to treat T1DM. The goal is sustained normoglycemia without the risk of hypoglycemia; in recent clinical trials, primary endpoints have been normalization of serum HbA1c as a marker of improved blood glucose control and the absence of hypoglycemic events. The benefits of islet allotransplantation over whole-organ transplant include avoidance of complications like graft thrombosis, anastomotic leaks, graft pancreatitis, cardiac complications associated with major surgery, as well as an expanded donor organ pool (donors with higher BMI have good islet yields but are avoided for whole-organ transplants). The disadvantages with islet allotransplants includes the loss of β-cell tissue during the isolation process and immediately after transplant, leading to the need of sequential islet infusions from two or more donors (according to CITR 2009 data, 26% of the recipients received a single infusion, 49% received two infusions, 23% received three infusions, and 2% received four infusions), and the exposure of higher concentration medications from blood delivered from the bowels by first-pass metabolism. Thus, some patients may benefit more from one or the other procedure.

Islet transplantation is considered an experimental treatment and as such is regulated by the U.S. Food and Drug Administration (FDA) under an Investigational New Drug application. Therefore, clinical trials and the production of the biological product (i.e., islets) are regulated by the FDA. Specifically, the FDA regulates the release criteria that are used to determine whether islets should be transplanted into a patient. Both safety (endotoxin levels, gram stain) and potency (insulin release index after glucose stimulation, viability, and immune-incompetent mouse bioassay) are assayed.

Patients with type diabetic mellitus for more than five years and meeting at least one of the following situations that persist despite intensive insulin management efforts (defined by monitoring glucose values at home at least three times each day and administering at least three insulin injections each day or insulin pump therapy, in close cooperation with an endocrinologist—i.e., at least three contacts during the previous 12 months) should be considered suitable candidates:

1. Metabolic lability or instability, characterized by two or more episodes of severe hypoglycemia (defined as an event with symptoms consistent with hypoglycemia in which the patient requires the assistance of another person, associated with a blood glucose measurements below 50 mg/dL or prompt recovery after oral carbohydrate, IV glucose, or glucagons administration) or two or more hospital admissions for diabetic ketoacidosis during the previous 12 months. Reduced awareness of hypoglycemia (defined as 4 > "R" responses on the hypoglycemia questionnaire or as clinical manifestation of hypoglycemia-associated autonomic failure)

2. Progressive secondary complications (defined by a [1] minimum of a three-step progression using the ETDRS grading system, or an equivalent progression as certified by ophthalmologist familiar with diabetic retinopathy; [2] autonomic neuropathy with symptoms consistent with gastroparesis, postural hypotension, neuropathic bowel or bowel or bladder, or persistent or progressive severe, peripheral, painful neuropathy not responding to usual management (e.g., tricyclic, gabapentin, or carbamezepin; or [3] progressive nephropathy, defined by a confirmed rise of at least 50 μg/min (72 mg/24 hours) of microalbuminuria over at least 3 months, beginning within the past 2 years, despite the use of an ACE inhibitors).

Islet autotransplantation is indicated in cases where severe chronic pain from chronic pancreatitis is treated with total pancreatectomy. Digested pancreatic tissue containing β-cells are infused into the portal vein during the same procedure. Islets in this case are not purified to minimize islet loss and time spent in the operating room. The disadvantage of using unpurified islets is that the higher volume of transplanted tissue can cause portal hypertension and inability to transplant the whole volume of digested pancreas, thus resulting in poorer glycemic control.

Islet Isolation and Transplantation

The method of islet isolation was described in 1988 by Dr. Ricordi et al. Cadaveric pancreas procurement for islets is similar to that of whole-organ transplantation. The total pancreatectomy procedure in pancreatitis patients differs from the standard procedure in that the vascular pedicle (splenic artery and splenic vein) is preserved until the graft can be completely removed. It is then flushed with cold preservation solution.

The procured pancreas is brought to the islet isolation laboratory. Extraneous tissue (lymph nodes, and fat) is trimmed off, and the duodenum and vessels are carefully removed from the graft. A solution of the digestive enzymes collagenase and protease is infused into the pancreatic ducts. Enzymatic digestion of the gland is combined with physical agitation to effectively dissociate the pancreatic tissue. This digested tissue (if <15 mL) may be directly transplanted into patients undergoing auto-islet transplantation following pancreatectomy.

Islets are purified for allotransplant recipients (or autotransplant recipients if the islet volume is >15 cc) by density gradient separation. This allows the islets (of lighter density) to be separated from the exocrine tissue. In general, 30% purity is required for allotransplantation. Allogeneic islets are cultured 24 to 36 hours following isolation to allow for lot-release testing, usually comprising glucose-stimulated insulin release, viability and purity assessment, islet enumeration, Gram stain, and measurement of endotoxin content.

Auto-Islet Transplantation

1. Total pancreatectomy
2. Reconstruction of gastrointestinal system
3. Intraportal islet infusion: In the Lab, the islet preparation is suspended in a tissue culture medium containing albumin and heparin (35–70 units/kg recipient body weight). In the operating room, the islet preparation is infused by gravity, monitoring the portal pressure. The infusion is halted if the pressure exceeds 22 mmHg and resumed when it is below 18 mmHg.

Allogeneic Islet Transplantation

1. Access to the portal vein: Percutaneous transhepatic catheterization by interventional radiology or minilaparotomy in the operating room with cannulation of an omental or mesenteric portal tributary vein; desobliteration of umbilical vein; and transjugular intrahepatic portosystemic shunt have also been described.
2. Intraportal infusion (as above)

Enrollment in Islet Allotransplantation Clinical Trials

The following inclusion and exclusion criteria are currently used by the Clinical Islet Transplantation (CIT) protocol CIT-07 (see www.isletstudy.org for details).

Inclusion Criteria

1. Male or female patients ages 18 to 65 years
2. Ability to provide written informed consent
3. Mentally stable and able to comply with the procedures of the study protocol
4. Clinical history compatible with T1DM with onset of disease at age younger than 40 years, insulin-dependence for 5 years or longer at the time of enrollment
5. Absent stimulated C-peptide (<0.3 ng/mL) in response to a mixed meal tolerance test measured at 60 and 90 minutes after the start of consumption

6. Involvement in intensive diabetes management under the direction of an endocrinologist, diabetologist, or diabetes specialist with at least three clinical evaluations during the 12 months prior to study enrollment
7. At least one episode of severe hypoglycemia in the 12 months prior to study enrollment
8. Reduced awareness of hypoglycemia (as defined by a combination of assessments of Clarke score, HYPO score, or glycemic lability) within the last 6 months prior to randomization

Exclusion Criteria

1. Body mass index (BMI) greater than 30 kg/m^2 or patient weight 50 kg or less
2. Insulin requirement of greater than 1.0 U/kg/day or less than 15 U/day
3. HbA1c greater than 10%
4. Untreated proliferative diabetic retinopathy
5. Blood pressure: SBP greater than160 mmHg or DBP greater than 100 mmHg
6. Measured glomerular filtration rate of less than 80 mL/min/1.73m^2
7. Presence or history of macro-albuminuria (>300 mg/g creatinine)
8. Presence or history of panel-reactive anti-HLA antibodies above background by flow cytometry
9. For female subjects: positive pregnancy test, presently breastfeeding, or unwillingness to use effective contraceptive measures for the duration of the study and 4 months after discontinuation. For male subjects: intent to procreate during the duration of the study or within 4 months after discontinuing or unwillingness to use effective measures of contraception
10. Presence or history of active infection (or with laboratory evidence thereof) including hepatitis B, hepatitis C, HIV, or tuberculosis (TB)
11. Negative screen for Epstein-Barr Virus (EBV) by IgG determination
12. Invasive asperigillus, histoplasmosis, or coccidioidomycosis infection within 1 year prior to study enrollment
13. Any history of malignancy with the exception of completely resected squamous or basal cell carcinoma of the skin
14. Known active alcohol or substance abuse
15. Baseline hemoglobin below the lower limits of normal at the local laboratory; lymphopenia, neutropenia, or thrombocytopenia
16. A history of Factor V deficiency
17. Any coagulopathy or medical condition requiring long-term anticoagulation therapy after transplantation (low-dose aspirin treatment is allowed) or patients with an international normalized value (INR) greater than 1.5

18. Severe co-existing cardiac disease, characterized by any one of these conditions:

    a. Recent myocardial infarction (within past 6 months)

    b. Evidence of ischemia on functional cardiac exam within the last year

    c. Left ventricular ejection fraction less than 30%

19. Persistent elevation (values >1.5 times normal upper limit) of liver function testes at the time of study entry

20. Symptomatic cholecystolithiasis

21. Acute or chronic pancreatitis

22. Symptomatic peptic ulcer disease

23. Severe unremitting diarrhea, vomiting, or other gastrointestinal disorders potentially interfering with the ability to absorb oral medications

24. Hyperlipidemia despite medical therapy

25. Receiving treatment for a medical condition requiring chronic use of systemic steroids, except the use of 5 mg or less of prednisone daily, or an equivalent dose of hydrocortisone, for physiological replacement only

26. Treatment with any anti-diabetic medication other than insulin within 4 weeks of enrollment

27. Use of any investigational agents within 4 weeks of enrollment

28. Administration of live attenuated vaccine(s) within 2 months of enrollment

29. Any medical condition that, in the opinion of the investigator, will interfere with safe participation in the trial

30. Treatment with any immunosuppressive regimen at the time of enrollment

31. A previous islet transplant

32. A previous pancreas transplant, unless the graft failed within the first week as a result of thrombosis, followed by pancreatectomy, and the transplant occurred more than 6 months prior to enrollment

Intensive Care Unit Management of Islet Transplant Patients

As mentioned above, islet transplantation is indicated in two groups of patients: those with auto-immune T1DM and those with chronic pancreatitis complicated by severe chronic pain that undergo total pancreatectomy followed by auto-islet transplantation.

Intensive care unit care is routine for patients undergoing total pancreatectomy and auto-islet transplantation. The risk of bleeding and complications associated with the gastrointestinal and biliary reconstruction is significant. In addition, these patients have a high tolerance to pain medication, so post-operative management of pain may necessitate continuous infusion of morphine analogs and/or ketamine. Continuous respiratory monitoring is indicated in these patients. Another major complication reported in this setting includes portal thrombosis during the first 7 days after infusion. Patients at risk for this (generally those with significant elevations of portal pressure following infusion) may need to be treated with systemic heparinization.

The CITR summarizes adverse event information in islet transplant recipients. The 6th Annual Report reported that 62% of the islet-only recipients experienced at least one adverse event during the first year post-transplant, whereas 44% experienced one or more serious adverse event (as defined by and reportable to the FDA, when the patient outcome is death, life-threatening, required hospitalization, caused disability or permanent damage, led to congenital anomaly or birth defect, or other serious/important medical events). Most common serious adverse events included neutropenia, elevated serum creatinine and elevated liver function tests, procedural hemorrhage, abdominal pain, pneumonia, portal vein thrombosis, diarrhea, or hypoglycemia. Of the adverse events reported in first year after first infusion for islet-only recipients, 32% were related to the immunosuppression therapy, and 27% were related to the infusion procedure.

The CITR reported nine deaths in islet allograft recipients. One case of viral meningitis 3 years after the last islet infusion possibly related to the immunosuppression. The other deaths resulted from drug toxicity (acute methadone and diphenhydramine), stroke, acute respiratory distress syndrome, pneumonia, diabetic ketoacidosis, atherosclerotic coronary artery disease, and one unknown.

Blood Glucose Control after Transplant and Metabolic Monitoring

The management of post-operative blood glucose is identical to that described for whole-organ pancreas transplantation.

Successful long-term islet allograft function is associated with the transplanted β-cell mass (>10,000 islet equivalent [IEQ]/kg body weight) lead to higher rates of graft function (as measured by C-peptide level) and early insulin independence in recipients with T1DM; however, following 1 year post-transplant, the insulin-independence rate declines for unclear reasons. In contrast, islet autograft recipients show a higher insulin-independence rate post-transplant, even if the estimated transplanted islet mass is less compared to islet allografts. This difference could be explained by donor factors (brain death), cold ischemia time, recipient allo-immune response, auto-immune recurrence, the presence of immunosuppressive drugs, and unknown factors.

Islet graft function can either be full, partial, or failed. Full islet graft function is defined by insulin independence; partial function by the use reduced doses of exogenous insulin in the presence of serum C-peptide; and failed if the patient is on a unchanged insulin regimen as compared with pretransplant requirements. Patients are monitored by serial post-transplant HbA1c levels together with glucose (or L-arginine)-stimulated C-peptide levels. The insulin-independent patients usually exhibit adequate C-peptide response (2 hours stimulated C-peptide levels ≥0.5 ng/mL) and Hb1Ac ≤7%.

Future Directions In Islet Transplant

The insufficient availability of human donors for islet transplantation creates opportunities for research in alternate sources of β-cell tissue. These include expansion of β cells, controlled differentiation of human embryonic stem cells into insulin-producing cells, or xenogeneic transplantation. The University of Pittsburgh recently joined a small number of research groups that provide rationale for clinical trials in islet xenotransplantation using genetically modified pigs as donors. Genetically engineered tissue may allow for improved engraftment, avoidance of cell death or injury, and also for local immunosuppression. Work is currently ongoing to optimize the combination of genetic modifications and to define safe and effective systemic immunosuppression in islet xenotransplantation.

Results from islet transplantation are steadily improving.; However, potent immunosuppression is still required. The development of immunological tolerance strategies would avoid allorejection and auto-immune-mediated recurrence of T1DM, as well as side effects and costs associated with immunosuppressive medicines. The hematopoietic cell transplant (HCT) has been developed to treat hematological malignancies; however, applying HCT to treat nonmalignant conditions has been impeded by graft-versus-host-disease. The establishment of mixed allogeneic chimerism (i.e., survival of both host and donor hematopoietic elements) can successfully achieve tolerance in mice, swine, and monkeys.

Another area of investigation is immune-isolation of islets within a semipermeable barrier to protect them from immunological rejection without the need for continued immunosuppression; this has been proposed for protecting islet cells. These immunobarrier devices utilize a semipermeable membrane designed to permit exchange of nutrients, glucose, and insulin with the host but exclude immunoglobulins, complement, and immunocompetent cells. Successful application of immune-isolation of islets has been demonstrated in small animals.

Significant advances have been made in all these areas in recent years and hold promise for future management options for patients with T1DM. Hopefully, several of these advances can be extended to also include patients with T2DM, then possibly impacting 25.8 million American children and adults (from the 2011 National Diabetes Fact Sheet; accessible on the Centers for Disease Control and Prevention website, www.cdc.gov).

Selected References

Shapiro AM, Lakey JR, Ryan EA, Korbutt GS, Toth E, Warnock GL, Kneteman NM, & Rajotte RV. Islet transplantation in seven patients with type 1 diabetes mellitus using a glucocorticoid-free immunosuppressive regimen. *NEJM*. 2000;343(4):230–238.

Chapter 23

Small Bowel and Multivisceral Transplantation

Guilherme Costa, Richard J. Hendrickson,
Jose Renan da Cunha-Melo, and Kareem Abu-Elmagd

Introduction

The intestine was one of the first solid organs surgeons attempted to transplant, but until 1990, only two patients survived isolated cadaveric intestinal grafts. For nearly three decades, the small intestine was considered forbidden from clinical transplantation because of associated massive lymphoid tissue, high antigenicity, and microbial colonization. With the revolutionary introduction of tacrolimus, FK506 (Prograf®, Astellas Pharma US, Deerfield, IL) in 1989, successful transplantation of human intestinal grafts alone or as a part of a composite visceral allograft became possible. With better survival outcomes and recognition by the United States Center for Medicare and Medicaid Services (CMS) in 2000, intestinal and multivisceral transplantation have been used more frequently for patients with irreversible gastrointestinal failure who can no longer be maintained on total parenteral nutrition (TPN) therapy or effectively treated for complex abdominal surgical disease.

Indications

Table 23.1 shows both surgical and nonsurgical causes of intestinal failure. Patients with surgical etiologies generally suffer from loss of bowel length after extensive resections for treatment of trauma injuries, volvulus, arterial or venous thrombosis, or repetitive resections for treatment of strictures and fistulas associated with Crohn's Disease, radiation enteritis, and adhesions. With the nonsurgical causes of intestinal failure the anatomic length and gross morphology of the intestine can be preserved such as in gastrointestinal pseudo-obstruction, Hirschsprung disease, and in absorptive problems, such as microvillus inclusion disease seen in the pediatric population.

Total parenteral nutrition is the standard of care for patients with intestinal failure who are unable to maintain a normal nutritional, fluid, and electrolyte balance through the gastrointestinal tract alone.

Table 23.1 Indications for Isolated and Composite Intestinal Transplantation

Nonsurgical	Surgical
Pseudo-obstruction	Gastroschisis
Intestinal atresia	Necrotizing enterocolitis
Microvillus inclusion disease	Volvulus
Intestinal polyposis	Trauma
Hirschsprung disease	Superior mesenteric artery thrombosis
Radiation enteritis	Crohn's disease
	Desmoid tumor
	Familial polyposis
	Gastrinoma
	GIST
	Budd-Chiari disease
	Intestinal adhesions
	Inflammatory bowel disease

Irreversible intestinal failure and complex abdominal visceral disease with failure of the currently available conventional therapeutic modalities, including TPN, are the prerequisites for the indication of intestinal and multivisceral transplantation. In October 2000, the CMS approved intestinal, combined liver/intestine, and multivisceral transplantation at centers of excellence as a standard of care for patients with irreversible intestinal failure who could not be maintained on TPN because of any of the following criteria: (a) TPN-associated liver injury, as manifested by jaundice or elevated liver tests, clinical findings (splenomegaly, varices, coagulopathy), history of stomal bleeding, or liver cirrhosis on biopsy; (b) loss of major venous access, defined by more than two thromboses in the great vessels (subclavian, internal jugular, or femoral veins); (c) frequent central line-related sepsis consisting of more than two episodes of systemic sepsis per year, or one episode of line-related fungemia associated with septic shock or acute respiratory distress syndrome; or (d) recurrent episodes of severe dehydration despite IV fluid management. Transplantation of the intestine, either alone or accompanied by other abdominal organs (liver, stomach, duodenum-pancreas, colon), may be lifesaving in this group of patients.

Pre-Transplant Evaluation

Referral for Transplantation

Patients with intestinal failure are commonly referred for transplantation after the development of life-threatening complications. Total parenteral nutrition and the short intestine are responsible for the development of

TPN/Short Gut syndrome associated liver failure. Late referral is associated with significantly higher morbidity and mortality among candidates waiting for combined liver/intestinal allografts compared to isolated small intestine transplant candidates. Data from the Intestinal Transplant Registry shows a significantly higher survival rate for patients who received transplants while waiting at home compared to patients who were hospitalized because of advanced disease. Patients dependent on TPN have chronic problems with central venous access. Patients with intestinal failure are particularly prone to infectious complications of their central venous catheter resulting from external contamination or secondary to translocations of microorganisms across a gut with inadequate barrier function. History of one or several episodes of line sepsis requiring treatment in an intensive care unit (ICU) is a rule. Infections caused by Gram-negative bacteria and fungus are common and are associated with high morbidity and mortality rates. These episodes of line sepsis contribute to further deterioration of the renal and hepatic functions. Vanishing of central venous access secondary to thrombosis is another common event observed in TPN-dependent patients.

Nutritional Assessment

An initial complete assessment of the patient nutritional status, including a thorough medical and surgical history, clinical examination, and biochemical markers, is performed. Failure to maintain the patient at their calculated ideal body weight without TPN or during weaning off TPN is a simple practical parameter indicating poor enteric functional reserve and indicative of irreversible gastrointestinal failure.

Gastrointestinal Tract

As part of the evaluation process, the gastrointestinal tract is studied from an anatomic and functional point of view. Radiological, endoscopic, and histological evaluation of the remaining hollow viscus and liver are conducted. Patients with history of gastrointestinal pseudo-obstruction require gut motility studies to define the extent of the disease and the etiology—whether myogenic, neurogenic, or mixed.

Hypercoagulable Status

Hematologic studies (Table 23.2) to rule out deficiencies of inactivator proteins of the cascade of coagulation, genetic mutations of coagulating factors, and the presence of thrombogenic antibodies are important in this highly complex population. In these patients, thrombogenic events are often the cause of their intestinal failure or they become hypercoagulable as a result of development of Short Gut syndrome.

Central Veins Assessment

Angiographic studies of the upper and lower central venous system are essential to document patency and guide placement of central venous accesses for TPN and IV hydration, more importantly for establishment of adequate venous access

Table 23.2 Work-Up for Hypercoagulation

Protein S

Protein C

Anti-thrombin III

Lupus anticoagulant antibody

Anti-cardiolipin antibody

Prothrombin gene mutation

DAPC resistance

Factor V Leiden

JAK2 Kinase mutation to rule out polycythemia vera

Flow cytometry for CD55 and CD59 to rule out Paroxysmal Nocturnal Hemoglobinuria

at the time of transplantation. The venogram in Figure 23.1 shows complete thrombosis of the right subclavian vein, brachiocephalic vein, and upper cava, and the computerized tomography (CT) shows large chest wall venous collaterals secondary to thrombosis of the major central veins. For patients requiring simultaneous replacement of the liver with the intestine, adequate central venous access above the diaphragm is imperative for volume resuscitation and transfusion of blood products during the anhepatic phase of the surgery. Alternative venous access techniques have been described for patients with vanishing of central venous access.

Visceral Angiogram

In patients with histories of complete vascular thrombosis, a complete visceral angiogram is mandatory to assess the extent of splanchnic vascular occlusion, including the arterial (superior mesenteric artery and celiac trunk) and portal (superior mesenteric vein, splenic vein, and portal vein) systems and is important to guide the type of visceral allograft needed. Hypercoagulable patients with diffuse thrombosis of the venous splanchnic system (Fig. 23.2) can become candidates for multivisceral transplant for treatment of liver failure and gastroesophageal variceal bleeding, rather than for intestinal failure. In these complex patients, isolated liver transplantation may not be feasible because of the technical failure to restore portal flow to the allograft caused by extensive portomesenteric thrombosis.

Liver Function

Evaluation of the degree of hepatic dysfunction (hyperbilirubinemia, transaminases abnormalities, hypo-albuminemia, thrombocytopenia, and coagulopathy), evidence of portal hypertension, status of the arterial perfusion to the liver, and the extension of liver disease by histology (bridging fibrosis or cirrhosis) are essential to determine the need for simultaneous replacement of the liver and intestine. Adequate specialized management of TPN can result in significant improvement of liver dysfunction, avoiding the need to replace the native liver.

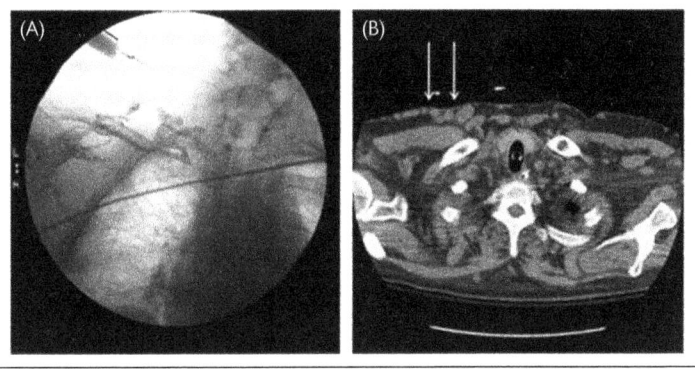

Figure 23.1. (A) Venogram showing central vein thrombosis: right subclavian vein, right brachiocephalic vein and upper cava. **(B)** CT showing intense venous collateralization at the subcutaneous tissue of the upper chest wall secondary the central veins thrombosis.

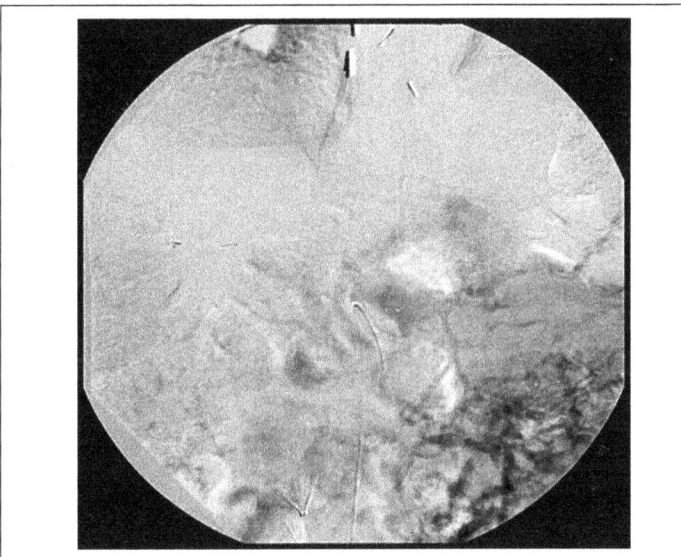

Figure 23.2. Superior mesenteric arteriogram with venous phase showing complete thrombosis of the porto-mesenteric venous system.

Renal Function

Renal function is studied because these patients normally present with histories of multiple admissions for dehydration and for line sepsis evolving with acute renal failure. In some instances, concomitant kidney transplantation is necessary.

Cardiovascular Function

Cardiac function evaluation starts with an electrocardiogram, transthoracic echocardiogram, or transesophageal echocardiogram (in cases of suspicious intracavitary thrombosis associated with central venous catheters). A heart stress test is requested for those who fall in the age group for high incidence of coronary artery disease or for those with histories warranting further heart evaluation. In select cases, a left heart catheterization is required to assess the extent of coronary artery disease. A right heart catheterization is required to measure pulmonary artery pressure when pulmonary hypertension is identified in the echocardiogram.

Pulmonary Function

Investigation of pulmonary status is completed with CT scan of the chest and pulmonary function test with arterial blood gas for those with previous histories of lung disease or smoking.

Further Evaluation

Further investigation of other systems depends on the patient's age, medical and surgical history, and nature of the gastrointestinal disorder.

In patients with histories of malignant disease and those at high risk for malignancies, serum markers for cancer (prostatic-specific antigen [PSA], alpha-fetoprotein [AFP], and carcinoembryonic antigen [CEA]) are requested.

Immunology

An immunological evaluation is performed, with double confirmation of the patient's ABO group, Human Leukocyte Antigen (HLA) typing, panel reactivity antigen (PRA), and the presence of anti-HLA class I and II antibodies by Luminex® assay. In patients with documented high levels of anti-HLA antibodies, a virtual cross-match is performed at the time of the organ offer to guide the decision-making process to accept that specific organ for the anti-HLA hypersensitized candidate. This virtual crossmatch is an attempt to reduce the incidence of antibody-mediated acute cellular and later graft loss secondary to chronic rejection.

Adrenal Function

A cortisol stimulation test is used to adequately assess adrenal gland function to assure an appropriate response to the intense surgical stress involved in transplantation. These patients often present with a history of chronic disease and have been taking long-term or intermittent exogenous corticosteroids. Also the correlation of liver cirrhosis with adrenal insufficiency is well established.

Psychological-Psychiatric Evaluation

A thorough psychiatric evaluation should address the patient's understanding of the magnitude and necessary commitment for this specialized surgical treatment, treat underlying psychological and psychiatric disturbances, and address issues related to pain control. Transdermal pain management is preferred.

Pre-Transplant Surgery

Some patients will require an exploratory laparotomy before transplant for control of abdominal sepsis, drainages of abdominal/pelvic collections, repair of intestinal fistulas, and surgical assessment of the remaining intestine's length and health. The control of abdominal infection previous to transplantation is paramount for the success of these challenging operations.

Listing for Transplant

A comprehensive multidisciplinary discussion involving case management staff, social workers, psychology/psychiatric staff, the pre-transplant nurse coordinator, gastroenterologist, immunologist, cardiologist, and transplant surgeons occurs to determine final acceptance and to list the patient for transplantation.

Care During the Waiting Period

During the pre-transplant evaluation and waiting periods, patients are closely followed. Total parenteral nutrition is frequently adjusted to optimize nutritional status, maintain adequate hydration, correct electrolyte abnormalities, and minimize TPN-induced liver dysfunction. Patients and caregivers are instructed about the management of central lines, ostomies, and tubes. Surveillance blood cultures are obtained periodically.

Contraindications for Transplantation

The contraindications for isolated intestine, liver-intestine, and multivisceral transplantation were primarily established based on historical experience with transplantation of other abdominal organs. These contraindications are either relative or absolute and include, but are not limited to, significant cardiopulmonary insufficiency, incurable malignancy, persistent life-threatening intra-abdominal or systemic infections, and severe immune deficiency syndromes. A history of gastrointestinal malignancy, the presence of resectable desmoid or stromal tumors, and an active abdominal infection at the time of referral should not be considered absolute contraindications for transplantation. In addition, loss of central venous access should not preclude transplantation, and age should not be considered a contraindication, unless it is associated with one or more of the prohibitive risk factors.

Management of the Transplant Candidate in the Intensive Care Unit

Intensive care of patients with intestinal and combined intestinal and liver failure presents major challenges that can be divided in two categories: (1) need for TPN and associated vascular access issues and (2) development of liver dysfunction. The most common reasons for admission to the ICU are sepsis associated with line infection, variceal bleeding with or without liver function decompensation, and severe dehydration. Because patients have been repeatedly exposed to multiple broad spectrum antibiotics and because the intestinal barrier is compromised, infections in patients with intestinal failure can be caused by multiresistant organisms. Fungal infections occur more commonly in these patients compared to the general population. Also, patients with liver failure have impaired immune responses. Impaired neutrophil and Kupffer cell oxidate burst function, and reduced complement levels have been documented.

Adrenal insufficiency with failure of the stress cortisol response is common in patients with history of long-term treatment with corticosteroids and in patients with acute and chronic liver failure. Adequate replacement of corticosteroids should be given as a bolus followed by maintenance doses. The combination of adrenal insufficiency, relative immune deficiency, and the intestinal transplant candidate's need for invasive procedures creates a high susceptibility to infection, sepsis, and shock.

Cardiac function in small intestine transplant candidates with liver disease is not normal, and one should have this fact in mind when managing septic shock. Patients with severe liver failure may have a baseline hyperdynamic state but a decreased contractile stress response. Both systolic and diastolic functions can be impaired. Resuscitation should be appropriately aggressive, with careful attention paid to signs of intravascular fluid overload, as patients may have concomitant Hepatopulmonary or Hepatorenal syndrome. Echocardiogram can be used to assess cardiac filling and function because invasive monitoring with a Swan-Ganz catheter can be precluded by the absence of a central venous access. In patients with advanced liver disease, albumin may be preferable to crystalloid as a resuscitation fluid to avoid worsening anasarca. High salt loads (e.g., normal saline) should be avoided in established liver disease.

The support of inotropes and vasopressors should be used if clinical signs suggest that the patient is intravascularly repleted. Early septic shock follows a vasodilatory pattern and may respond to vasopressor agents. Again, the possibility of adrenal insufficiency should be considered in patients with septic shock unresponsive to catecholamines and treated if necessary.

The removal of the infected line is imperative, and the placement of a temporary central access is necessary for resuscitation maneuvers, antibiotics, and TPN. When the infection is cleared, a new central venous access should be established. Normally the interventional radiology group places this definitive access with the assistance of ultrasound and angiography.

The patient's nutritional status should be maintained by TPN and the infusion of lipids held when the patient is sedated with lipidic medications and when sepsis is secondary to fungemia.

Isolated intestinal transplant candidates may have mild, reversible liver disease. On the other hand, patients waiting for a combined liver-intestine or multivisceral transplant may manifest overt liver failure. Coagulopathy, portal hypertension with ascites and hepatomegaly, variceal bleeding, hypo-albuminemia, hyperbilirubinemia, hyperammonemia with hepatic encephalopathy, Hepatorenal syndromes, and Hepatopulmonary syndromes may all be seen in this population of patients.

Mechanical ventilation should be promptly considered when indicated. However, all efforts should be made to achieve early and safe extubation to avoid problems associated with intravenous sedation, respiratory muscle deconditioning, and ventilator-associated pneumonia. Pharmacological neuromuscular blockage to facilitate artificial ventilation should be discouraged as often as possible, because these malnourished and deconditioned patients will require a very prolonged neuromuscular function recovery period after extubation, which can preclude them from undergoing transplantation. Extra caution should be used when tracheostomy is needed, because of problems associated with bleeding and infection.

The indications for drainage of ascites must be weighed against the risk of infection. The development of catheter-associated peritonitis can definitively contraindicate a transplant with a dismal outcome. The treatment of coagulopathy can be achieved with administration of clotting factors (fresh frozen plasma [FFP], cryoprecipitate, platelets). It may be impossible to normalize the coagulation studies; rather, therapy should be guided by clinical evidence of bleeding. The transfusion of large volumes of blood products should be avoided in these patients with impaired renal and heart functions. In case of severe or recurrent bleeding, plasma exchange (plasmapheresis) and the use of recombinant factor VII have been successful in correcting coagulopathy without fluid overload. However, these measures should be carefully applied to patients with a hypercoagulable status.

Transplantation

Types of Intestinal Allografts

Patients with gastrointestinal failure are candidates for an isolated small intestine, small intestine-pancreas, liver-intestine, modified multivisceral, or a full multivisceral transplant. The type of intestinal allograft (Fig. 23.3) required by each patient is dictated by the anatomic and functional status of each solid and visceral abdominal organ. The entire length or a segment of the large bowel may be included in the allograft, particularly in those patients who could benefit from a pull-through operation or any reconstructive surgical procedures. An en bloc or heterotopic kidney allograft is also transplanted in patients with established or imminent renal failure.

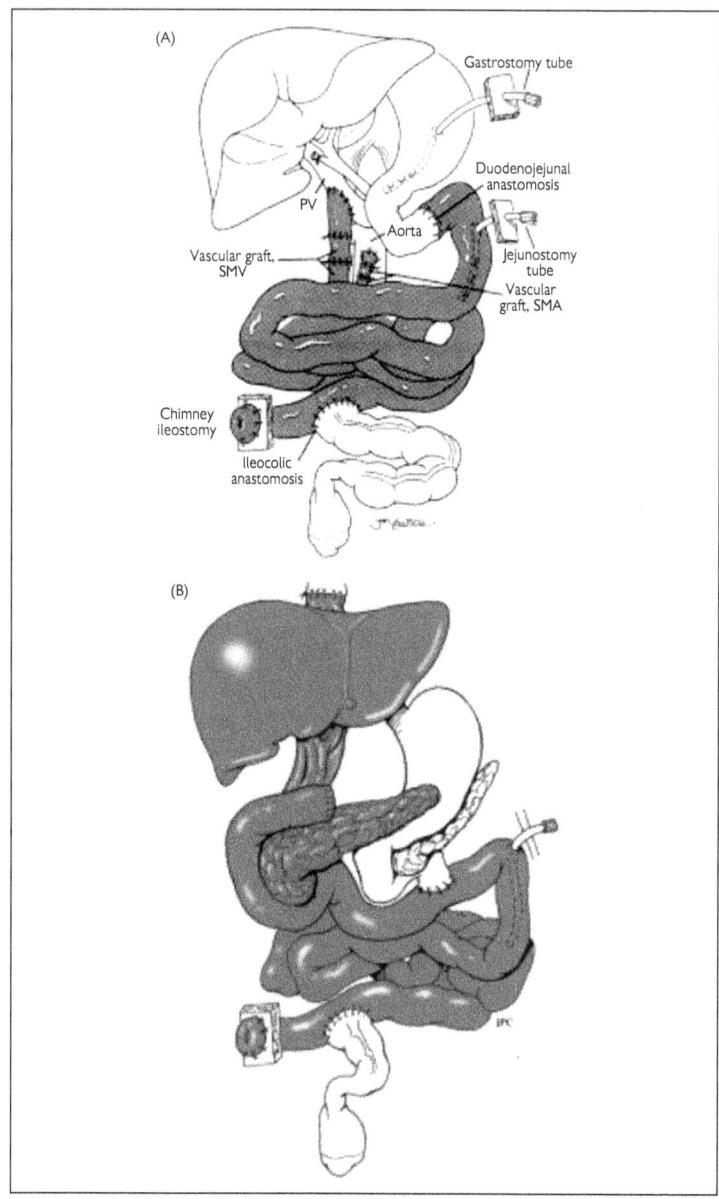

Figure 23.3. Types of intestinal allografts. **(A)** Isolated small intestine; **(B)** Liver-intestine; **(C)** Modified-multivisceral; **(D)** Multivisceral. For **(A)**, **(B)**, and **(D)**, the allograft is the dark part. For **(C)** allograft is the white part.

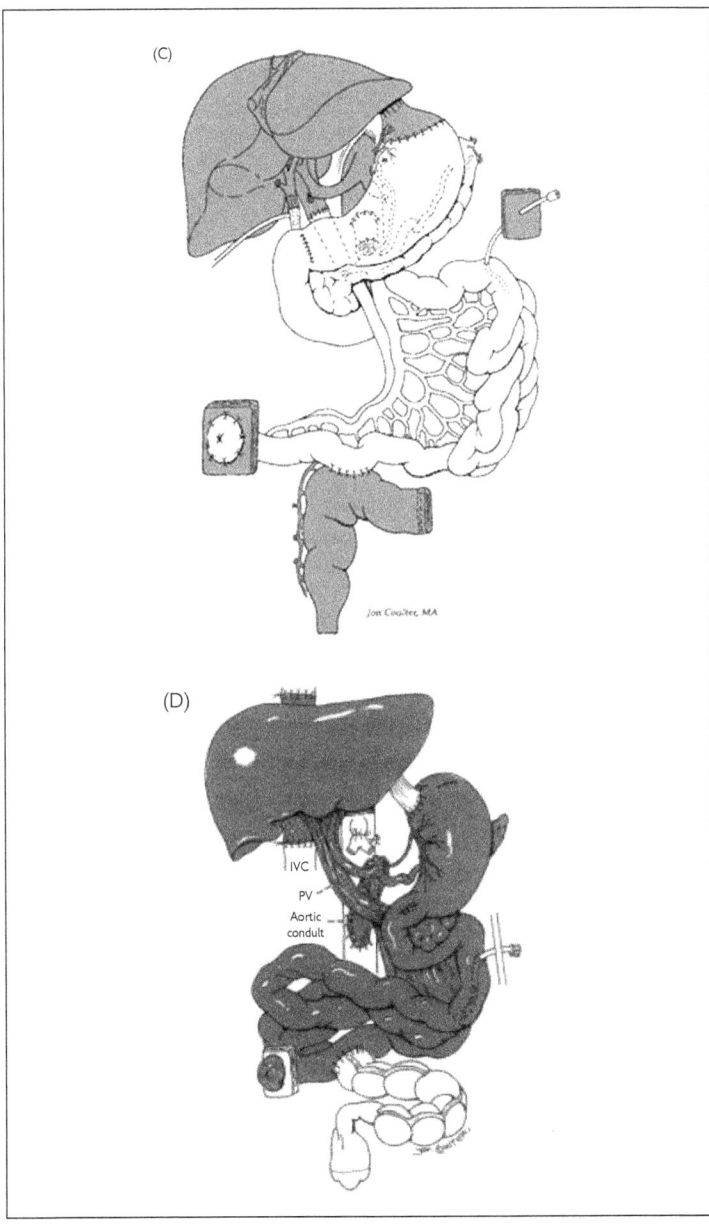

(C)

Jon Coulter, MA

(D)

IVC
PV
Aortic
conduit

Figure 23.3. (*Continued*)

Intra-Operative Management

As part of the pre-transplant evaluation, a member of the Transplant Anesthesia Team examines the patient, reviews the work-up, and determines a strategy for anesthesia. Status of the central venous access, cardiovascular status, and overall medical condition are taken in consideration.

The duration and complexity of the surgical procedure and the intensity of the anesthesia team's peri-operative care will be determined by the modality of intestine-containing allograft to be transplanted. An isolated intestine transplant normally involves less surgical dissection, and patients normally present with better overall nutritional status and liver function, as well as with more preserved heart and lung functionality. On the other hand, patients requiring a modified multivisceral, liver-intestine, or full multivisceral allograft with or without a concomitant kidney allograft will require significantly longer operative procedures, with major intravascular volume changes, metabolic derangements, transfusion of large volumes of blood products, and coagulopathies.

Because the surgical procedure can be very lengthy, special attention is paid to adequately positioning and protecting the different segments of the patient's body to avoid such undesirable complications as foot droop, pressure sores, stretching of brachial plexus, compression of ulnar and fibular nerves, and compartment syndrome of upper or lower extremities. Also, it is not uncommon for these patients to have severely decreased subcutaneous fat and muscle mass, allowing the direct contact of bone prominences with the surgical table, making adequate padding a necessity. A warming pad is placed over the cushion pads of the surgical table, and upper and lower body warming devices are also used.

External defibrillation pads for pacing or defibrillation should be placed for prompt action in case of a cardiac arrhythmia or cardiac arrest during the reperfusion phase.

The anesthesia team's required anesthesia and monitoring equipment for these patients consists of an anesthesia machine with a volume and pressure-controlled ventilator, capnography, mass spectroscopy bispectral index (BIS) monitor, EKG, blood pressure cuff, direct arterial blood pressure monitors, pulse oximeter, transesophageal echocardiogram (TEE), thromboelastogram (TEG), rapid infusion system, pulmonary artery catheter, and continuous cardiac output monitor. The use of a blood salvaging system is not professed in intestinal transplantation because of the high risk of abdominal contamination in patients with history of multiple surgeries, enteric fistulas, abdominal infections, and abscesses.

General anesthesia is normally induced through a peripheral venous access or, more commonly, through the central venous access being used for parenteral nutrition. This indwelling central line, which was used for TPN and hydration before the transplant, is then no longer used during the surgery because of the high risk of bacterial/fungal colonization. It is removed in the operating room before or right after completion of the operation. A radial arterial line is placed under local anesthesia before the induction of general anesthesia. The pre-operative venogram is reviewed before entering the operating room and is used to guide the placement of two large-bore central lines. Eight and a half or nine French introducers are placed for volume and medication administration and pulmonary artery catheterization. In patients with vanishing of the central veins caused by thrombosis, general anesthesia is induced with administration of medications via the arterial line, and the surgeon obtains venous access inside of the abdominal cavity through catheterization of one or both gonadal veins or inferior mesenteric vein. Thrombosis of the major central veins precludes the placement of a pulmonary artery catheter and TEE is used to assess the patient's volume status and myocardial function. A second arterial line should be placed in one of the femoral arteries for direct arterial blood pressure monitoring and blood sampling. A nasogastric tube and a Foley catheter are ordinarily placed. Ureteral stents are indicated in patients with histories of multiple abdominal surgeries, abdominal or pelvic irradiation, previous urinary tract surgery, or retroperitoneal tumors.

Patients presenting for any modality of small intestine transplant commonly suffer from delayed gastric emptying, and rapid sequence induction should be used to facilitate a safe endotracheal intubation. General anesthesia is maintained with a combination of inhalant anesthetic in an air-oxygen mixture, intravenous narcotics, benzodiazepines, and muscle relaxants.

Broad spectrum prophylactic antibiotics are administered at induction of anesthesia and throughout the procedure: aztreonam (2 g every 8 hours), vancomycin (1 g every 12 hours), or linezolid (600 mg every 12 hours) for patients allergic to vancomycin, metronidazole (1 g at induction and 500 mg every 8 hours thereafter), and liposomal amphotericin B (5 mg/Kg every 24 hours).

Preconditioning using lymphoid-depleting agents rATG (Thymoglobulin®, Genzyme, Cambridge, MA) or alemtuzumab (Campath-1H, ILEX, Cambridge, MA) is started at induction of anesthesia and infused over 4 to 6 hours and completed before reperfusion of the allograft. Premedication with acetaminophen (650 mg orally), diphenhydramine (25 mg intravenously), and methylprednisolone (1 g intravenously) is necessary. A second dose of methylprednisolone (1 g intravenously) is given when the allograft is brought to the surgical field for implantation.

Potassium containing intravenous solutions is avoided and parenteral nutrition containing potassium is interrupted upon admission to the hospital for transplant. The patient's hydration and blood sugar is maintained with a solution of dextrose and sodium chloride until reaching the operating room. Potassium level is maintained below 4 mEq/L to avoid hyperkalemia at the moment of allograft reperfusion, which could predispose the patient to cardiac arrhythmias and cardiac arrest.

Continuous monitoring of cardiac output, central venous pressure (CVP), mean pulmonary artery pressure (PAP), pulmonary capillary wedge pressure (PCWP), mixed venous oxygen saturation (SvO_2), right ventricular ejection fraction, right ventricular end-diastolic volume, and core temperature is routinely performed.

The surgical procedure can be divided in three distinct phases: dissection of the remaining diseased organs and preparation of the allograft's arterial inflow and venous outflow (stage I), vascular anastomosis (stage II), and after reperfusion of the allograft, gastrointestinal reconstruction (stage III). During the dissection phase, the grade of surgical adhesions, intensity of the portal hypertension associated or not with partial or complete portomesenteric venous thrombosis, and thrombocytopenia secondary to hypersplenism or secondary to the effects of the rATG or Alemtuzumab can be responsible for significant blood loss and coagulopathy. Also during this phase, partial clamping of the abdominal aorta in a supraceliac or infra-renal position will cause dampening of femoral arterial line's wav form and should be communicated by the transplant surgeon to the anesthesia team. The unclamping of this vessel should also be communicated because of the possibility of systemic blood pressure dropping when the lower part of the recipient's body is reperfused. In the second phase, the allograft is brought to the surgical field, the vascular anastomoses are constructed, and the organs are reperfused. The reperfusion period will be discussed in detail later in this chapter. During the third phase of the surgical procedure, the patient is expected to hemodynamically stabilize, improve metabolically, and achieve adequate hemostasis. During this period, the gastric (in a modified multivisceral or multivisceral transplant), biliary (in a modified multivisceral transplant with removal of the native pancreas and duodenum), and the proximal and distal intestinal anastomoses, as well as the feeding jejunostomy and ileostomy, will be created.

To maintain hemodynamic stability during the surgical procedure, adequate hydration with a balanced administration of 0.9% sodium chloride and 5% albumin in a 50:50 ratio should be accomplished. A transplant of an intestine-containing allograft could take 12 to 15 hours and requires several hours of dissection, leaving behind a large bare surface in the abdominal cavity. Because of changes in capillary permeability secondary to release of endotoxins from intra-abdominal foci of infection and from the surgical manipulation of diseased viscera, there is an intense extravasation of fluid to the third space (extravascular space) manifested by anasarca and rapid exsudation and accumulation of intra-abdominal fluid. The continuous communication between the surgical and anesthesia teams is fundamental to discuss the necessary changes in fluid resuscitation. Most of the blood loss occurs during stage I of the surgical procedure; the goal of replacement therapy for RBC transfusion is to achieve a hematocrit level of 28% to 30%. This allows for optimal oxygen delivery, avoidance of increased viscosity with higher hematocrit levels, and increased survival in post-operative critically ill patients.

Patients requiring isolated intestine transplant or any other modality of an intestine-containing allograft frequently behave as hypercoagulables despite normal traditional clotting studies such as prothrombin time, activated partial thromboplastin time, international normalized ratio, and platelet count. This was confirmed by a study from our institution using TEG. A comprehensive hypercoagulable work-up is performed at the pre-operative evaluation to guide our pre-, intra-, and post-operative management of this patient population. Thromboelastography is a test of whole-blood coagulation (Fig. 23.4). It allows the measurement of the initial formation of fibrin strands, measured by the reaction time (r) within 10to 14 minutes. Clot formation rate (α) or the

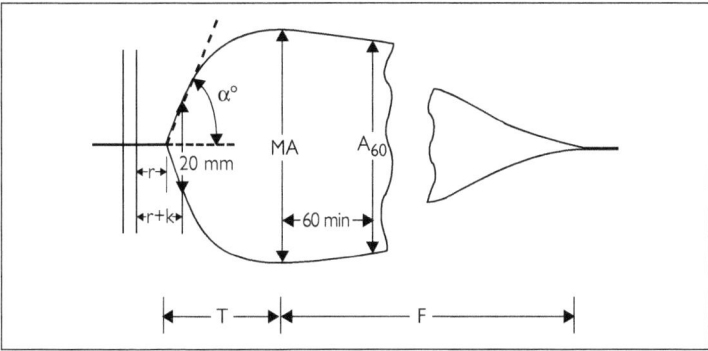

Figure 23.4. Thromboelastograph tracing. A_{60}, amplitude 60 min after MA; A_{60}/MA x 100, whole-blood clot lysis index greater than 85%; α, clot formation rate (53°–67°). F, whole-blood clot lysis time greater than 300 min; MA, maximum amplitude (59–66); r, reaction time (10–14min); r + k, coagulation time (13–20 min); T, time to MA.

speed at which a clot forms is normally 53° to 67° and is a function of fibrinogen and platelets. Normal coagulation is represented by a progressive increase in amplitude, reaching maximum amplitude (MA) of 59to 68 mm. Maximum amplitude is a function of the elasticity of the blood clot. The value is increased by improved platelet function, fibrinogen, and factor XIII (fibrin stabilizing factor). A significant reduction in r time and a significant increase in α-angle have been observed in patients requiring a modality of intestine-containing transplant. The TEG should, in conjunction with a minimum coagulation profile (prothrombin time, activated partial thromboplastin time, international normalized ratio, and platelet count) should guide the transfusion of blood products or the administration of anti-fibrinolytic agents as epsilon aminocaproic acid. Because of the fact of most of the patients are hypercoagulable, a very conscious replacement of blood products such as FFP, cryoprecipitate, and platelets is recommended to prevent catastrophic complications as intracavitary heart clots or thrombosis of vascular anastomosis. One common side effect of the infusion of the antilymphocyte preparation used in our pre-conditioning protocol (rATG or Campath) is thrombocytopenia; prompt and pre-emptive correction of this disturbance is paramount to avoid uncontrollable surgical bleeding in an extensively dissected abdomen.

The precise monitoring of hemodynamic parameters demonstrates a significant elevation in the cardiac output, mean PAP, CVP, and PCWP immediately after reperfusion of the allograft. In addition, systemic vascular resistance decreases 20% from baseline approximately 2 hours after incision, reaching a low (40% below baseline) throughout the remainder of the procedure. Hypotension, with mean arterial pressure less than 60 mmHg, defined as "postreperfusion syndrome," can be found in up to 47% of the recipients of an intestine-containing allograft. This incidence of Post-Reperfusion syndrome is higher compared to liver transplantation. The use of vasoactive agents such as epinephrine, norepinephrine, and dopamine can be necessary to support blood pressure in patients with significant vasodilatation. It is not uncommon for some patients to be kept on continuous infusion of a low dose of norepinephrine during the surgical procedure, which is easily weaned off during the first hours at the ICU.

Close attention should be paid to electrolyte composition, mainly potassium and calcium levels. The serum potassium, as stated before, should be kept below 4 mEq/L. In patients with renal insufficiency or renal failure, a pre-operative session of hemodialysis can be necessary because potassium-lowering agents such as insulin-glucose infusions, sodium bicarbonate, and albuterol inhalation would not be efficient to achieve normokalemia and to reduce total corporal potassium. In some cases, intra-operative hemodialysis should be considered for clearance and/or ultrafiltration. The practice of evacuation through the infrahepatic inferior vena cava of the first passage blood from the allograft prevents an overload of potassium and other inflammatory mediators retained on the allograft during the period of cold ischemia. The monitoring of ionized calcium is imperative, mainly in patients requiring large volumes of blood transfusions to avoid coagulopathy, arrhythmias, and myocardial depression. Hypomagnesemia and hypophosphatemia are also not uncommon in Short Bowel syndrome and should be properly corrected.

The intra-operative lactate curve normally steadily increases until reperfusion and then starts decreasing to reach a normal range after the first hours of recovery at the ICU. Some patients requiring a modality of intestine-containing allograft present with some grade of liver disease secondary to the effects of TPN, absence of hepatotrophic hormones delivered to the liver in a set of Short Gut syndrome, or secondary to sequel of ischemic hepatitis and behave intra- and post-operatively with a slow metabolic recovery attested by the lactate curve.

A continuous infusion of intravenous tacrolimus (1 mg/24 hours) is started after reperfusion of the allograft.

After reperfusion, continuous infusion of prostaglandin E1 (PGE$_1$, Asprostadil®) is started at the dose of 0.1 to 0.6 μg/Kg/h to increase the blood flow to the intestinal allograft as an attempt to reduce ischemia-reperfusion injury, minimizing platelet adhesion to the vascular endothelium. Because PGE$_1$ can cause hypotension, this medication is not started until the patient's blood pressure is normal without the need for vasoactive agents.

After obtaining hemostasis of the vascular anastomosis, the surgeons proceed with the gastrointestinal anastomosis. For patients receiving an isolated small intestine or en bloc intestine-pancreas, the proximal anastomosis will be performed in between the recipient's duodenum or proximal jejunum to the donor's jejunum. For those receiving a modified multivisceral or a full multivisceral allograft, the proximal anastomosis is created in between the stump of native stomach and the fundus of the allograft stomach. A pyloroplasty is also necessary, because of vagal denervation, to prevent gastric outlet obstruction. The distal anastomosis is then created in between the distal ileum allograft and the remaining segment of native large intestine, leaving a chimney segment which is exteriorized as an ileostomy to serve as access to surveillance endoscopies and biopsies of the allograft mucosa. In patients with previous proctocolectomies, the ileum is exteriorized as a definitive end ileostomy. The creation of a feeding jejunostomy is the last surgical step before proceeding with abdominal wall closure. In this group of patients, poor status of the abdominal fascia secondary to multiple previous abdominal surgeries frequently precludes the closure of the muscle layer, and closure of the skin is the only option. Finally, the patient is transferred to the ICU.

Post-Transplant Care in the Intensive Care Unit

For recipients with pre-transplant liver failure, post-operative care is similar (although more intense) to that provided for isolated liver transplant recipients. Recipients of isolated small intestine transplants who have stable liver function usually have a more routine initial ICU course.

Immunosuppression

Table 23.3 presents immunosuppression regimens used at the University of Pittsburgh from 1990 to 2011. Currently, alemtuzumab (Campath-1H, ILEX, Cambridge, MA) is used as the lymphoid-depleting agent, and the post-transplant immunosuppression strategy is tacrolimus monotherapy with avoidance, when possible, of maintenance steroid therapy. An intravenous dose of tacrolimus is started after reperfusion in the operation room to achieve a 12-hour trough level of 10 to 15 ng/mL by the third post-operative day. The same level is aimed for in the first 3 post-operative months, after which levels of 5 to 10 ng/mL are sought. A variable course of methylprednisolone, or more commonly hydrocortisone, is added in patients with positive T/B cell lymphocytic cross-match and those who develop Serum Sickness syndrome, adrenal insufficiency, allograft rejection, and graft-versus-host reaction. Highly HLA-sensitized patients may be required to enroll in a protocol using an anti-B-cell medication such as the proteasome-inhibitor bortezomib, (Velcade®, Millenium Pharmaceuticals, Cambridge, MA).

Table 23.3 Intestinal Transplantation: Immunosuppression Regimens by Era at the University of Pittsburgh
Years medications
May 1990—May 1994 Tacrolimus (T)/steroids (S)
January 1995—May 1998 T/S/Cyclophosphamide
May 1998—April 2000 T/S/Daclizumab
April 2000—June 2001 T/S/Daclizumab + ex vivo allograft irradiation
June 2001—August 2003 Anti-lymphoid preparation + ex vivo allograft
Irradiation + donor bone marrow augmentation
August 2003—present Anti-lymphoid preparation/T/±S

Ventilatory Management

Radiography of the chest should be performed upon admission to the ICU to confirm the position of the endotracheal tube, central lines, and Swan-Ganz catheter. The goal of ventilator management is early extubation. Isolated intestine recipients have better overall reserve and normally are able to be extubated on the same day of the transplant or on the first post-operative day. Decreased lung function, post-operative graft status, sepsis, inability to close the abdominal wall, presence of diaphragmatic weakness, and paralysis are factors to be considered when planning weaning off ventilatory support. The need to return to the operative room to complete the surgical procedure, to perform a second look, or to review the hemostasis are indications to keep the recipient on artificial ventilation. Pain management is a serious complicating factor for the process of weaning off artificial ventilation, because many patients with chronic diseases have been on long-term pain medications and appropriate control of pain to allow deep breathing can be difficult to obtain. After extubation, the respiratory therapist team should implement a hyperinflation protocol to avoid atelectasis, pneumonia, and need for re-intubation. Treatments with nebulized bronchodilators and hourly exercises with the incentive spirometer should be ordered, with the head of the bed elevated to 40 degrees. The patency and correct functioning of the nasogastric tube is assured at least three times a day to prevent a full stomach followed by vomiting and catastrophic aspiration pneumonia.

Hemodynamic Profile

Careful management of the central lines, Swan-Ganz catheter, and arterial lines is particularly important in these patients with poor venous access and diseased peripheral arteries. The loss of venous or arterial access can compromise transplants and potentially create a life-threatening situation where no access can be obtained.

The hemodynamic parameters monitored in small intestine recipients are CVP, arterial blood pressure, and urinary output. In those in whom the liver was replaced, a pulmonary catheter is placed in the operating room for continuous monitoring of cardiac output, pulmonary arterial pressure, end diastolic volume index, and mixed venous oxygen saturation. If a vasoactive medication is necessary in the operating room, starting with a small dose of norepinephrine and titrating to a minimum necessary dose is preferred. The most common scenario is for the patient to be weaned off vasopressor support promptly after admission to the ICU. Rarely, this class of medication is maintained longer than 24 hours. If, for some reason, a second vasoactive medication should be started, then vasopressin is to be considered. Proper fluid resuscitation should be done before starting infusion of vasoactive medications.

A continuous infusion of PGE1 (alprostadil, Prostin VR® Pediatric, Pfizer) at small doses of 0.2 μcg/Kg/hour titrated to a maximum dose of 0.6 μg/Kg/hour is started at the operating room or at the ICU as soon hemodynamic stability is achieved. The dose is titrated up if the blood pressure tolerates. The vasodilator and anti-platelet aggregation properties of alprostadil aim to protect the microvasculature of the recently reperfused allograft.

Infection Control (See Chapter 9)

Coagulopathy

Post-operative coagulopathy should be judiciously addressed. Because of the extent of surgical dissection necessary to perform the transplant, the consumption of coagulation factors continue in the post-operative period and a preemptive correction of the thrombocytopenia and of the depletion of coagulating factors is justified. Overcorrection of the coagulopathy, on the other hand, can be harmful for an allograft with fresh vascular anastomosis and with a possible micro-angiopathy secondary to the ischemia-reperfusion injury. A platelet count above 75,000 platelets/microliter is normally enough to maintain post-operative hemostasis. In highly HLA-sensitized patients, transfusion of HLA-matched platelets can be the only option to achieve an adequate count of circulating platelets. Low platelet count can be caused by the anti-lymphoid preparation used in the pre-conditioning or can reflect an intense inflammatory process caused by rejection of the allograft. If transfusion of clotting factors becomes necessary, then cryoprecipitate is preferred to FFP because of the higher concentration of these factors in a significantly lower volume. In recipients of multivisceral allografts, transfusion of cryoprecipitate twice or three times a day can be necessary in the first 2 days post-operatively.

Adrenal Function

Patients who do not continue corticosteroids after the peri-operative period should have a cortisol stimulation test repeated at post-operative day 5 to assert the capacity of the adrenal gland to respond to needs around the transplant period. A normal response to the ACTH stimulation test during the pre-transplant evaluation does not guarantee an adequate adrenal adaptation to the stress after the transplantation. An abnormal cortisol stimulation test should be followed by adequate replacement therapy, preferentially with hydrocortisone sodium succinate.

Neurological Function

Abnormal mental functions interfering with weaning off the ventilator or changes in mental functions after the extubation should raise concerns of toxemia caused by infectious processes or increased circulating cytokines secondary to allograft rejection. Toxicity of medications, mainly of the calcineurin inhibitor agent tacrolimus and of antibiotics, should not be underestimated as causes of changes in mental status.

Metabolic Profile

Isolated small intestine recipients with normal liver reserve develop a minimal metabolic derangement during transplantation. Patients with some grade of liver injury can present with metabolic acidosis that normalizes in the first 24 hours of admission to the ICU. Liver-intestine or multivisceral allograft recipients show a transient elevation of transaminases and usually correct the metabolic acidosis before leaving the operating room.

Renal Function

Adequate intra-operative hydration prevents acute kidney injury, and worsening of renal function in the immediate post-operative period is infrequent. In case of acute renal failure, continuous veno-venous hemodialysis (CVVHD) is preferable to intermittent hemodialysis, because of less aggressive fluid and electrolytes shifts in a short period of time and with more efficient fluid removal in a 24-hour period.

The patient's hydration status should allow adequate heart filling pressures and a proper perfusion of the tissues. Overhydration will interfere with the gas exchange in the lungs and result in a high CVP with venous congestion of the allograft, delaying the recovery of ischemia-reperfusion injury.

Nutrition

Moderate-to-severe malnutrition is commonly seen in patients with intestinal or intestinal and associated liver failure. Treatment with corticosteroids potentiates the catabolic status, and prompt nutritional intervention is started in the post-operative period to prevent further nutritional deterioration. Parenteral nutrition is resumed normally on post-operative day 1, and enteral feeding is started if the ostomy is healthy, non-edematous, the first small intestine mucosal biopsy does not show findings compatible with rejection, and signs of intestinal function are evident. An elementary enteral formula is normally started on post-operative day 7. Oral intake is started if the patient tolerates a full enteral feeding without a nasogastric tube. Early referral of patients for transplantation frequently allows faster recovery and oral intake without need for enteral feeding.

Management of Complications

Graft Rejection

Clinically, intestinal allograft rejection may be asymptomatic or present with fever, abdominal pain, distension, nausea, vomiting, or with increased or decreased ostomy output. The ostomy may appear normal or lose its normal velvety appearance and become edematous, friable, ulcerated, or become congested with a dusky color. Histologically the rejection is graded by the degree of epithelial damage. In mild rejection, epithelial cell apoptosis leads to epithelial cell loss within the deep crypts. In moderate rejection, more severe crypt damage with crypt loss is observed. Severe rejection leads to denuded mucosa. Regeneration occurs by epithelialization over the surface of a lamina propria devoid of crypts (Fig. 23.5). Acute rejection occurs in approximately 50% of patients receiving an anti-lymphoid preparation as a preconditioning agent. Mild allograft rejection responds to an IV bolus of methylprednisolone and optimization of tacrolimus levels in most of the cases. A bolus of methylprednisolone followed by a steroid taper is the initial treatment for moderate rejection. Cases of moderate rejection resistant to steroids or cases of severe rejection are treated with a lymphoid-depleting preparation rATG (Thymoglobulin®, Genzyme, Cambridge, MA) or

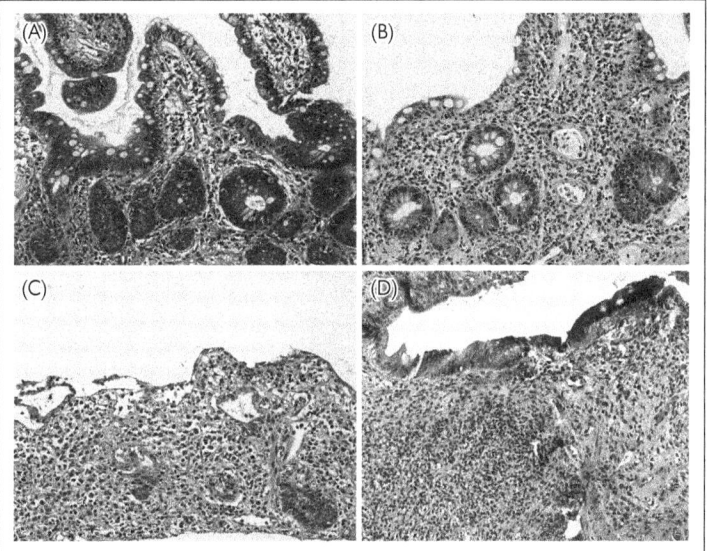

Figure 23.5. Mild rejection **(A)** characterized by cell apoptosis in the crypts. Moderate rejection **(B)** with confluent apoptosis and crypt injury. Severe rejection **(C)** showing denuded mucosa and cryptopenia. Regenerative mucosa **(D)** with intense epithelial cell proliferation.

alemtuzumab (Campath-1H, ILEX, Cambridge, MA). Highly HLA-sensitized recipients with known anti-HLA donor-specific antibodies may be better treated with steroids, and a combination of immunosuppressant drugs such as polyclonal intravenous immune globulin IVIg (Gammagard®, Baxter, Westlake Village, CA) at the dose of 2 g/Kg and bortezomib (Velacade®, Millenium Pharmaceuticals, Cambridge, MA) at the dose of 1.3 mg/m² of body surface area.

Chronic rejection of the intestinal allograft is documented in about 15% of patients. Concomitant rejection of the liver allograft in composite grafts has also been seen but at a lower rate. Liver-containing allografts (liver-intestine, multivisceral) experience a significantly better chronic rejection-free survival rate compared to liver-free isolated intestine and modified multivisceral allografts. Clinical presentation may include weight loss, chronic diarrhea, intermittent fever, abdominal pain, and gastrointestinal bleeding. Histologically, villous blunting, focal ulcerations, epithelial metaplasia, and scant cellular infiltrates are present in the endoscopic mucosal biopsies. Full-thickness intestinal biopsies show obliterative thickening of intestinal arterioles.

Pulmonary Complications

Almost invariably, intestinal transplant recipients leave the operating room with some degree of fluid overload. This situation is more likely to occur in the recipients of liver-containing allografts, as those recipients are in worse general status before the transplant and endure surgeries of longer duration. Adequate diuresis should be administered to properly address pulmonary edema if present. Figure 23.6 shows chest CT scans of a patient with Acute Respiratory Distress syndrome and severe pulmonary edema.

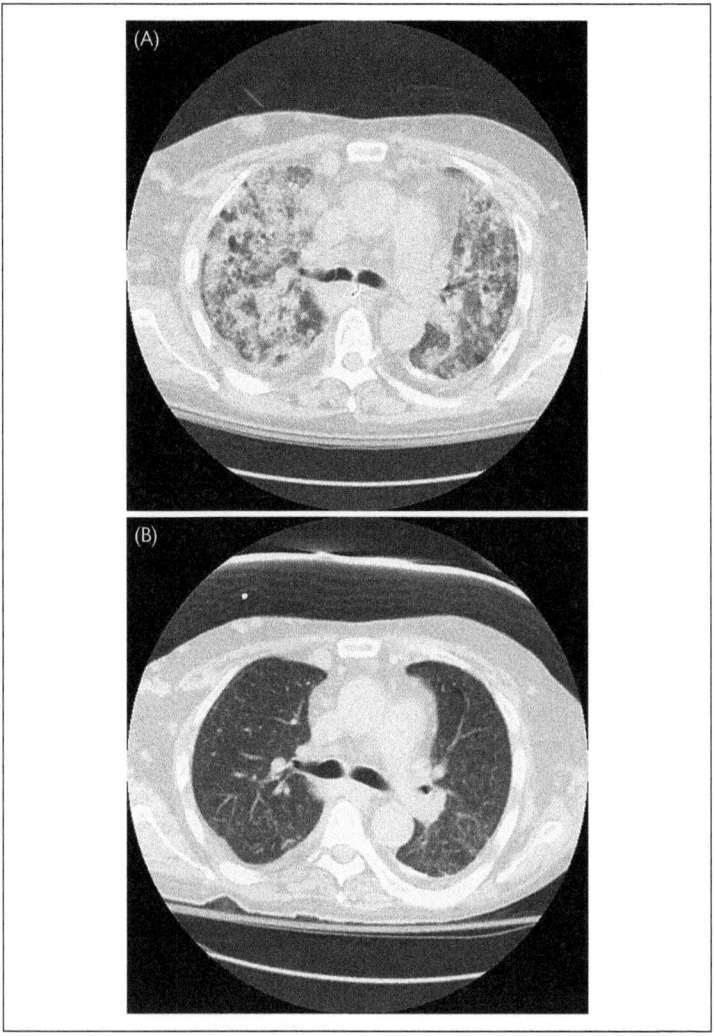

Figure 23.6. Chest CT scans showing **(A)** severe Acute Respiratory Distress syndrome and pulmonary edema treated successfully with CVVHD. **(B)** Follow-up CT scan 8 days later.

Patients with well-established pulmonary hypertension are cleared for transplantation if their mean pulmonary artery pressure is below 35 mmHg. In the post-operative period, these patients are monitored closely to avoid fluid overload and decompensation of right heart function.

Failure to extubate in a timely manner will significantly increase the chances of ventilator-associated pneumonia in a patient with decreased muscle mass and heavy immunosuppression.

Biliary Complications

With the modification in donor technique allowing preservation of the donor duodenum and entire pancreas with maintenance of the hepatopancreaticobiliary system, biliary and pancreatic complications from leaks and strictures from anastomoses have been avoided. However, a group of these patients have shown signs and radiological evidence of abnormal biliary tree. Ampullary dysfunction of a denervated allograft can be the cause of this problem, which can be solved with a percutaneous transhepatic cholangiographic approach and balloon dilatation and/or via endoscopic retrograde cholangiopancreaticogram with stenting or papilotomy.

In modified multivisceral allografts, continuity of the biliary tract is re-established, either via a duct-to-duct anastomosis or via a Roux-en-Y biliodigestive anastomosis. In the patients, biliary tract complications (i.e., leakages and obstructions) can occur.

Infection

Infectious complications continue to cause significant morbidity and mortality after intestinal transplantation. However, current immunosuppressive modifications have decreased the incidence of life-threatening bacterial complications, and fungal and viral infections are the main source of morbidity.

Fungal infections are more common after heavy treatment for rejection, extensive usage of antibiotics, intestinal leaks, and multiple surgical explorations. Prophylactic and active treatment of fungal infections has been achieved successfully because of the availability of new effective medications, including Liposomal Amphotericin B, Caspofungin, and Voriconazole.

Post-Transplantation Lymphoproliferative Disorder

With less aggressive immunosuppression, the incidence of PTLD has significantly decreased to less than 5% in the adult population. Mortality related to PTLD has decreased despite recipient partial lymphoid depletion. Risk factors for PTLD are the intensity of the immunosuppression, recipient age (children are more susceptible), and splenectomy. The clinical presentation of PTLD may vary from asymptomatic findings at routine endoscopy, Epstein-Barr virus enteritis and systemic symptoms, bleeding, lymphadenomegaly, or tumors. The treatment includes reduction of immunosuppression, antiviral therapy, monoclonal anti-CMV immunoglobulin, (Cytogam®, CSL Behring AG, Bern, Switzerland), anti-CD20 monoclonal antibody rituximab (Rituxan® Roche, Basle, Switzerland), and chemotherapy.

Cytomegalovirus Infection

The current incidence of cytomegalovirus (CMV) infection is 7%. Cytomegalovirus-polymerase chain reaction (PCR) assay is used for early detection and follow-up treatment for new infection or viral re-activation. Clinical presentation is usually with enteritis. Successful treatment is obtained in the majority of cases. Intravenous ganciclovir is used for 2 weeks prophylactically around the transplant and for treatment when necessary. Also, monoclonal anti-CMV immunoglobulin is given as an adjunct to ganciclovir for the treatment of active disease. A CMV-positive donor graft transplanted into a CMV-negative recipient is a significant risk factor for CMV disease, but monitoring of CMV-PCR with preemptive therapy has allowed the successful use of CMV-mismatched organs.

Graft-versus-Host Disease

Five percent of adults develop some grade of graft-versus-host-disease (GVHD) diagnosed by histopathological criteria and confirmed by immunohistochemical studies showing visable evidence of donor cell infiltration into the lesions or by flow cytometry detecting elevated donor cell chimerism in peripheral blood. The treatment consists of optimization of immunosuppression and limited steroid therapy. Interestingly, total donor-derived multilineage complete chimerism was documented in four adult recipients of liver-containing grafts in our institution.

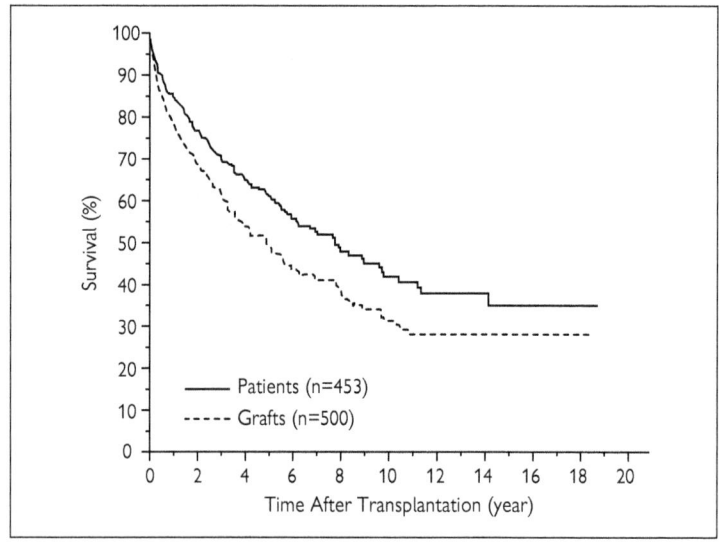

Figure 23.7. Kaplan-Meier patient and graft survival for the Pittsburgh experience from May 1990 to November 2008.

Outcomes

Survival Rates at Our Institution

Patient and graft survival are shown in Figure 23.8. The causes of graft loss are primary nonfunction (1% of the transplanted grafts), technical complications (4%), allograft rejection (20%), GVHD (1%), infection (11%), PTLD (3%), and others (8%). Liver-intestine allografts had the best long-term engraftment. (Fig. 23.8) With isolated small intestine allografts, early transplantation defined by less than 12 months of previous TPN therapy was associated with better survival: 57% at 5 years and 50% at 10 years (Fig. 23.9).

Worldwide Survival Rates

Data from the Intestine Transplant Registry show that a total of 2611 transplants were done worldwide to the year 2011. Seventy-nine centers have performed small intestine transplants, and 35 are currently active. From the total of transplants, 1148 (43.9%) were isolated small intestine, 845 (32.4%) were liver-small intestine, and 619 (23.7%) were multivisceral. Figure 23.10 shows the worldwide survival by graft type.

Currently there are 1341 (51.3%) patients alive worldwide, including adults and children. Among the 1148 patients alive, 813 are adults, and 158 (19.4%) were transplanted at the University of Pittsburgh. Among the 528 children alive, 139 (26.3%) were transplanted at the University of Pittsburgh.

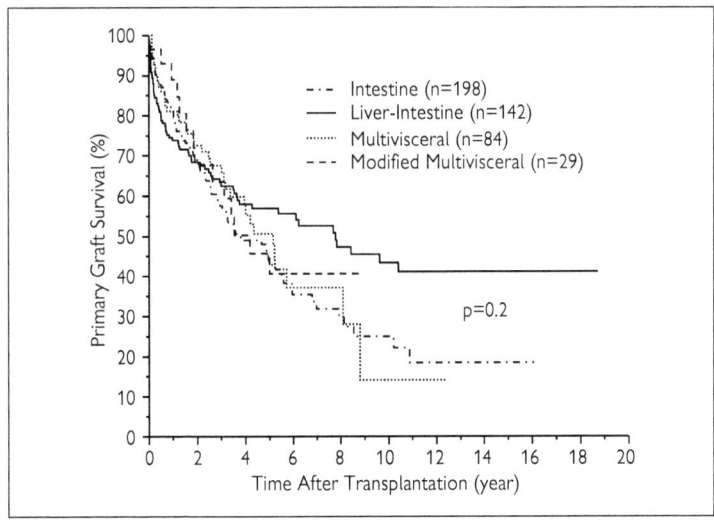

Figure 23.8. Kaplan-Meier primary graft survival curve according to age and type of visceral transplant.

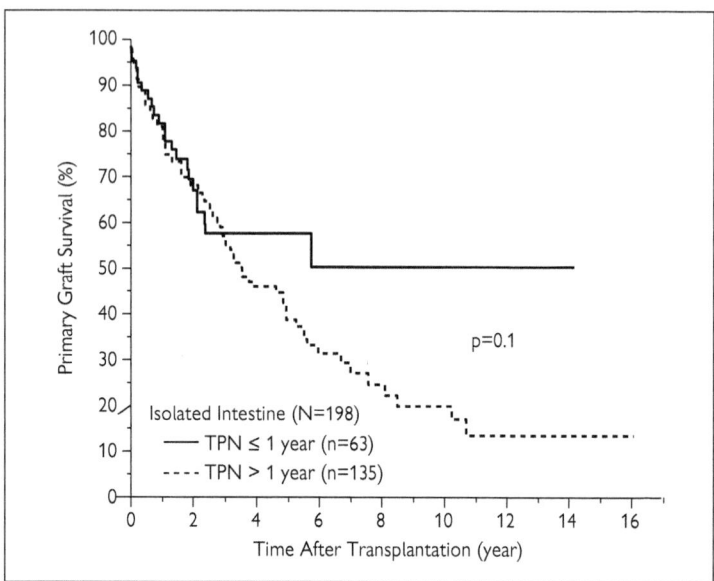

Figure 23.9. Kaplan-Meier survival of the primary intestine only allografts according to the duration of TPN before transplantation.

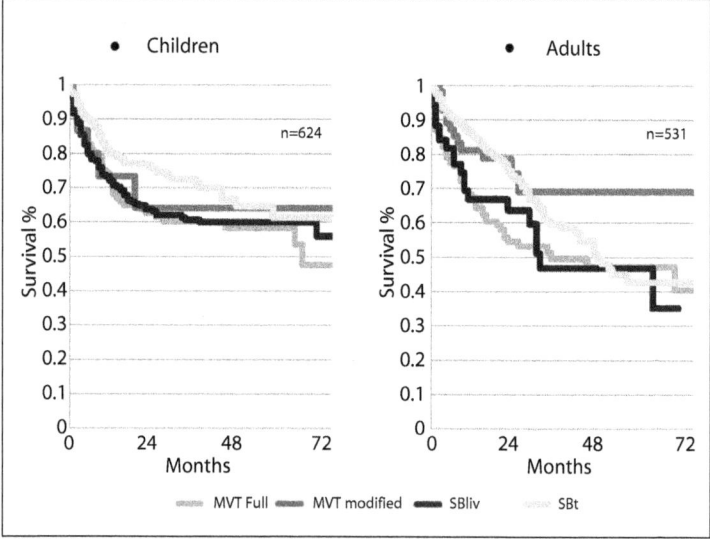

Figure 23.10. Kaplan-Meier survival according to type of visceral allograft for the World Experience (2006–2011).

Data from the Intestine Transplant Registry.

Selected References

Abu-Elmagd, KM, Mazariegos G, Bond G, et al. Intestinal transplantation: current status and future considerations. *Am J Gastroenterology* 2006;101:307.

Abu-Elmagd, KM, Costa G, Bond GJ, et al. Five Hundred Intestinal and Multivisceral Transplantations at a Single Center. *Major Advances With New Challenges. Ann Surg* 2009; 250(4):567–581.

American Gastroenterology Association (AGA). American Gastroenterological Association Medical Position Statement: Short bowel syndrome and intestinal transplantation. *Gastroenterology* 2003;124:1105–1110.

Index

"f" indicates material in footnotes and "t" indicates material in tables.